LIPEDEMA SOLUTION

NAVIGATING COMPRESSION THERAPY, DIET, AND SURGICAL OPTIONS FOR EFFECTIVE MANAGEMENT

BY

DR. ELVIRA S. GRAVES

TABLE OF CONTENTS

1. TABLE OF CONTENTS
2. Disclaimer
3. Introduction
4. Part I: The Science of Lipedema
5. Chapter 1: Lipedema: Defining the Disorder, Tracing Its Origins, and Understanding Its Anatomy and Physiology
6. Chapter 2: Stages and Types of Lipedema
7. Chapter 3 — Causes and Risk Factors of Lipedema
8. Chapter 4 — Lipedema vs. Other Conditions

9. Part II: Non-Surgical Management
10. Chapter 5 — The Role of Compression Therapy
11. Chapter 6 — Nutritional Strategies for Living Better with Lipedema
12. Chapter 7 — Exercise and Physical Therapy
13. Chapter 8 — Liposuction for Lipedema
14. Chapter 9 — Post-Surgical Care

15. Part III: Living with Lipedema
16. Chapter 10 — Psychological Impact and Support
17. Chapter 11 — Lifestyle Modifications
18. Chapter 12 — Patient Stories and Case Studies
19. CONCLUSION

Disclaimer

Copyright © by Dr. Elvira S. Graves 2024.
All rights reserved.
Before this document is duplicated or reproduced in any manner, the publisher's consent must be gained. Therefore, the contents within can neither be stored electronically, transferred, nor kept in a database. Neither in Part nor full can the document be copied, scanned, faxed, or retained without approval from the publisher or creator.

Introduction

From Confusion to Clarity

In the relentless quest for health and well-being, knowledge is more than just power—it is the ultimate form of empowerment. For millions of women worldwide, the journey toward understanding their own bodies has been marred by confusion, dismissal, and silence. **"Lipedema Solution: Navigating Compression Therapy, Diet, and Surgical Options for Effective Management"** is more than just a book; it is a compass designed for those navigating the turbulent and often lonely waters of a condition shrouded in mystery and misinformation.

For too long, Lipedema has been the "invisible disease," hidden in plain sight. This book serves as your definitive guide through the complexities of a disorder that has been historically misunderstood by society and frequently misdiagnosed by the medical community. Here, we move beyond the frustration of unanswered questions and step into a structured pathway of care, validation, and hope.

Understanding Lipedema: Beyond the Surface

To manage Lipedema, one must first deeply understand it. Lipedema is a chronic, progressive fat disorder, widely believed to be hereditary, that manifests as a symmetrical and disproportionate accumulation of adipose tissue. This accumulation typically occurs in the legs, hips, and buttocks, and frequently affects the arms. However, this is not "normal" fat.

Unlike standard obesity, Lipedema fat is often painful to the touch, bruises easily, and is resistant to traditional diet and caloric restriction.

One of the defining characteristics explored in these pages is the "two-body syndrome"—where the upper torso may remain slender while the lower body accumulates significant mass. Crucially, we distinguish Lipedema from **Lymphedema** (a problem with the lymphatic drainage system, though the two can coexist) and general obesity.

In this book, we will delve into the pathophysiology of the condition. You will learn about the **"Cuff Sign"** (where fat stops abruptly at the ankles or wrists), the hormonal influences of puberty, pregnancy, and menopause that often trigger the condition, and the fibrotic changes in the tissue that create the characteristic "nodular" texture under the skin.

The Critical Importance of Early Diagnosis

Time is a vital factor in the management of Lipedema. An early diagnosis can be the defining line between manageable maintenance and facing a lifetime of severe mobility issues and orthopedic complications. Tragically, the average patient often waits decades for a correct diagnosis, enduring years of "gaslighting" where they are told to simply "eat less and move more."

We underscore the critical nature of recognizing the early signs—such as heavy legs, unexplained bruising, and texture changes—before the condition progresses to later stages (Lipo-Lymphedema). This book outlines specific diagnostic criteria and provides a roadmap for how to speak to medical professionals. We aim to shorten the "diagnostic odyssey," equipping you with the terminology and clinical evidence needed to advocate for the care you deserve immediately, not years down the line.

Debunking Myths and Misconceptions

Lipedema is fraught with damaging myths that lead to profound stigma and inadequate care. The psychological toll of being judged as "lazy" or "gluttonous" when suffering from a metabolic disorder is immense. We dispel these myths methodically and scientifically.

- **The Diet Myth:** We dismantle the notion that Lipedema is simply a result of poor self-control. We explain why Lipedema fat does not burn off through standard caloric deficits.
- **The "Cosmetic" Myth:** We challenge the insurance and medical perspective that treating Lipedema is purely for aesthetic reasons, highlighting the debilitating pain and mobility loss involved.
- **The Untreatable Myth:** Perhaps most importantly, we refute the idea that nothing can be done. While there is currently no "cure," there are highly effective management strategies.

This book aims to dismantle the misconceptions that have hindered progress and understanding for so long, replacing judgment with physiological fact.

A Holistic Approach: The Pillars of Management

This book does not rely on a single solution. Instead, it offers a multi-modal approach to treatment. We navigate the three main pillars of Lipedema management:

1. **Conservative Therapies:** We provide a deep dive into Complete Decongestive Therapy (CDT), the science of Manual Lymphatic Drainage (MLD), and the crucial role of compression garments—explaining the difference between flat-knit and circular-knit fabrics and how to find the right fit for your stage.
2. **Nutritional Interventions:** We explore anti-inflammatory protocols (such as RAD, Keto, or Mediterranean variations)

specifically tailored to reduce the systemic inflammation and fluid retention associated with Lipedema.

3. **Surgical Options:** We offer an unbiased look at Lipedema-sparing liposuction (WAL, TAL, etc.). We discuss who is a candidate, what the recovery looks like, and realistic expectations for outcomes regarding pain reduction and mobility improvement.

Exclusive Benefits for the Reader

What sets this book apart is its comprehensive, patient-centered focus. By reading this, you will gain:

- **Expert-Driven Insight:** Knowledge synthesized from leading specialists in lymphology, vascular surgery, and nutrition.
- **Actionable Protocols:** Not just theory, but practical, daily routines for skin care, donning compression, and lymphatic exercises.
- **Surgical Transparency:** Detailed guidance on vetting surgeons, understanding risks, and preparing for the financial and physical aspects of surgery.
- **Empathetic Support:** A collection of shared stories and experiences from the "Lipedema Sisters"—women who have walked this path and found ways to thrive.
- **Self-Advocacy Tools:** Templates and checklists to take to your doctor's appointments to ensure you are heard and treated correctly.

Your Path Forward

By choosing **"Lipedema Solution,"** you are not just purchasing a resource; you are investing in a lifeline. You are choosing to reject the silence and shame that often accompanies this condition. This book offers hope, clarity, and a tangible path forward. Whether you are newly diagnosed or have been managing symptoms for decades, this guide is your partner in reclaiming agency over your body and your life.

Part I: The Science of Lipedema

Chapter 1: Lipedema: Defining the Disorder, Tracing Its Origins, and Understanding Its Anatomy and Physiology

Introduction: The Mystery of the "Heavy Legs"

Imagine a woman who exercises four times a week. She tracks her macronutrients diligently, maintains a caloric deficit, and drinks plenty of water. Over six months, she loses weight from her face, her waist, and her bust. Her ribs become visible, and her collarbones sharpen. Yet, her legs remain exactly the same—heavy, column-like, and painful to the touch. For decades, this woman might have been told by doctors that she was simply "obese" or that she was "lying" about her food intake. She might have been prescribed diuretics that did nothing or aggressive diet plans that only resulted in metabolic damage.

This is the quintessential Lipedema experience.

Lipedema is not obesity. It is not a cosmetic flaw, and it is certainly not a failure of will. It is a distinct, chronic, and progressive medical condition. Specifically, it is an **adipofascial disorder**, characterized by a symmetrical and disproportionate accumulation of diseased fatty tissue, primarily in the lower extremities (legs, hips, buttocks) and often in the arms. Crucially, this condition spares the hands and feet, creating a distinct "cuff" effect where the swelling stops abruptly at the ankles or wrists. It is a condition of contradictions: the upper body may be anorexic while the lower body is morbidly obese; the skin may feel soft but is incredibly painful to the touch.

In this chapter, we will strip away the confusion. We will define Lipedema not just by what it looks like, but by what is happening beneath the skin. We will trace its historical origins, explore the genetic and hormonal triggers, and take a deep dive into the anatomy and physiology that separates Lipedema fat from regular adipose tissue.

The Origin Story: A History of Misunderstanding

While Lipedema feels like a "new" discovery to many—often due to the explosion of awareness on social media—it was actually identified over 80 years ago.

In **1940**, Drs. Edgar V. Allen and Edgar A. Hines Jr. at the Mayo Clinic first identified a specific syndrome involving "fat legs" and fluid accumulation. By **1951**, alongside Dr. Lester E. Wold, they published their seminal paper formally coining the term **"Lipedema"** (originally spelled *Lipoedema* in European literature). They described it as a condition characterized by "large legs due to the subcutaneous deposition of fat and the accumulation of fluid."

Despite this early identification, Lipedema largely disappeared from American medical curricula for the latter half of the 20th century. It remained a focus of study primarily in Germany and Austria, where lymphatic research was more advanced. This geographical gap in knowledge explains why so many patients in the US and UK today struggle to find a doctor who recognizes the name, let alone knows how to treat it.

The Epidemiology: Hiding in Plain Sight

How common is it? The statistics are staggering. Current research estimates that Lipedema affects approximately **11% of the post-pubertal female population** globally. To put that in perspective, that is roughly one in every nine women. This makes Lipedema more common than Type 1 Diabetes or Rheumatoid Arthritis, yet it receives a fraction of the research funding and medical attention.

The condition is almost exclusively found in females. While there have been rare case reports of men developing Lipedema, these usually occur in the presence of severe hormonal imbalances (such as liver failure or testosterone deficiency). This stark gender divide points us directly to the root cause: **Hormones.**

Tracing the Origins: Genetics and Hormones

The exact etiology (cause) of Lipedema is multifactorial, but two pillars stand out: genetic predisposition and hormonal turbulence.

1. The Genetic Link

"I have my grandmother's legs."

If you have Lipedema, you have likely said or heard this phrase. There is a strong hereditary component to the disorder. Research suggests an X-linked dominant or autosomal dominant inheritance pattern with sex limitation. This means the gene is passed down through families, but the "switch" to turn the condition on is usually only flipped in females. If your mother, aunt, or grandmother struggled with heavy, painful legs, easy bruising, or mobility issues, they may have been undiagnosed Lipedema patients. Recognizing this pattern is crucial not just for your own validation, but for identifying the condition in younger generations (daughters and nieces) before it progresses.

2. The Hormonal Storm

Lipedema is inextricably linked to estrogen. The onset of the disease almost always correlates with periods of significant hormonal flux:

- **Puberty:** The most common time for onset. A teenage girl may notice her legs getting "thick" or "chunky" regardless of her activity level.
- **Pregnancy:** Many women report a rapid exacerbation of symptoms during or immediately after pregnancy.
- **Menopause:** The shift in hormones during perimenopause often triggers a flare-up, where the disease progresses from a purely cosmetic concern to a painful, mobility-limiting condition.
- **Gynecological Surgery:** Procedures involving the ovaries or uterus can sometimes act as a trigger.

This hormonal connection suggests that Lipedema tissue possesses unique estrogen receptors, causing the fat cells in these specific areas to react differently than fat cells elsewhere in the body.

Anatomy and Physiology: What Lies Beneath?

To manage Lipedema, you must understand the "enemy." Lipedema is not just "extra fat." It is a complex dysfunction of the adipose tissue (fat), the lymphatic system, and the vascular system.

1. The Adipose Tissue (The Fat Cells)

Normal weight gain typically involves **hypertrophy**—where existing fat cells get bigger. Lipedema involves both hypertrophy and **hyperplasia**—where the fat cells actually increase in number.

Furthermore, the structure of the fat is different. In the early stages, the skin may look smooth, but as the condition progresses, the subcutaneous tissue undergoes fibrotic changes.

- **Nodular Texture:** If you palpate (feel) the legs of a Lipedema patient, you will not feel smooth, squishy fat. You will feel nodules. These range from the size of rice grains or peas (in Stage 1) to walnuts (Stage 2) or even fist-sized masses (Stage 3). This is often described as feeling like a "bag of beans" or "Styrofoam balls" under the skin.
- **Inflammation:** Lipedema fat is metabolically active in a negative way. It releases inflammatory cytokines (signaling proteins) that create a state of chronic, low-grade inflammation in the legs.

2. The Vascular System (The Blood Vessels)

One of the hallmarks of Lipedema is **capillary fragility**. The tiny blood vessels (capillaries) within the Lipedema fat are weak and prone to breaking. This leads to the tell-tale symptom of **easy bruising**. A patient might wake up with a large bruise on her thigh and have no memory of bumping into anything. This is because the expanding fat tissue stretches the capillaries to their breaking point, and the vessel walls themselves are structurally compromised.

3. The Lymphatic Connection (The Fluid)

For years, it was debated whether Lipedema was a lymphatic disorder. We now know it is. While the large lymphatic vessels might function normally in the early stages, the **micro-lymphatics** (the tiny vessels responsible for draining fluid from the tissue spaces) are overwhelmed.

Here is the mechanism: The enlarged fat cells compress these tiny lymphatic vessels. Additionally, the capillaries are "leaky," allowing more fluid to escape into the tissue than normal. The lymphatic system cannot keep up with this increased load. The result is **edema** (swelling). This fluid is rich in protein, and when protein-rich fluid sits in the tissue, it causes inflammation and triggers the body to lay down scar tissue (**fibrosis**). This fibrosis locks the fat in place, making it even harder to lose.

4. The Pain Mechanism

Why does it hurt? The pain in Lipedema is likely a combination of:

- **Tissue Pressure:** The expanding fat cells and fluid exert immense pressure on the nerve endings.
- **Inflammation:** The inflammatory chemicals irritate the nerves.
- **Hypoxia:** The overgrown tissue may not get enough oxygen, leading to a state of hypoxia (oxygen starvation), which is painful.

Clinical Presentation: The Signs and Symptoms

Diagnosing Lipedema is primarily clinical, meaning it relies on a physical exam and patient history rather than a blood test. A savvy clinician looks for the following "Checklist of Evidence."

The Physical Appearance

- **Disproportionate Distribution:** The classic "pear shape," but exaggerated. A woman might need a size XS top and XL pants.
- **The "Cuff" or "Bracelet" Sign:** This is a key differentiator. The swelling typically stops at the ankles (or wrists), creating a sharp demarcation. The feet usually remain normal (unless secondary Lymphedema has set in).
- **Symmetry:** Unlike Lymphedema, which often starts in one leg, Lipedema usually affects both legs equally.
- **Fat Pads:** Common distinct deposits include pads of fat on the insides of the knees (causing gait issues) and on the outer thighs (saddlebags).

The Sensory Experience

- **Pain and Tenderness:** "The cat walking on my lap hurts." This hypersensitivity is a major red flag.
- **Heaviness:** A sensation that the legs are "made of lead" or "filled with cement," especially by the end of the day.
- **Cold Skin:** The affected areas often feel cooler to the touch than the trunk of the body, indicating poor blood flow through the adipose tissue.

The Diagnosis: Navigating the Medical Maze

Because there is no single biomarker for Lipedema, diagnosis is often a process of exclusion—ruling out other conditions like Dercum's Disease, general obesity, or primary lymphedema.

The Physical Exam

A provider should palpate the tissue to check for the "bean-bag" texture. They will check for **Stemmer's Sign**.

- **The Test:** The doctor attempts to pinch and lift the skin at the base of the second toe.
- **The Result:** If the skin *can* be pinched and lifted, Stemmer's Sign is **Negative**. This usually indicates Lipedema (as the feet are spared). If the skin is thick, tight, and cannot be lifted, Stemmer's Sign is **Positive**, which indicates Lymphedema. *Note: In advanced Lipedema (Stage 4 or Lipo-Lymphedema), the sign may become positive as the lymphatics fail completely.*

Imaging and Tests

While not strictly necessary for diagnosis, these tools help confirm the condition and assess severity:

- **Ultrasound:** Can visualize the thickness of the subcutaneous fat and detect the characteristic "snowstorm" pattern of Lipedema tissue.
- **Lymphoscintigraphy:** A nuclear medicine scan that maps the flow of lymph fluid. It helps determine if the lymphatic system is functioning or impaired.
- **DEXA Scan:** useful for differentiating between lean mass and fat mass, highlighting the disproportionate accumulation in the legs.

The Impact: The Cost of Living with Lipedema

We cannot define this disorder without acknowledging its profound impact on the human experience. Lipedema is a thief—it steals mobility, confidence, and mental peace.

1. Physical Disability

As the fat lobules grow, particularly on the inner thighs, they force the legs apart. This alters the patient's gait, leading to **valgus deformity** (knock-knees). The misalignment puts tremendous strain on the knee and hip joints, often leading to premature osteoarthritis. Many Lipedema patients end up needing knee replacements, but surgeons may refuse to operate due to their BMI, unaware that the "obesity" is actually a connective tissue disease.

2. The Psychological Toll

The mental health impact of Lipedema is severe. Years of failed dieting lead to a damaged relationship with food. Eating disorders—ranging from anorexia to binge eating—are tragically common as patients try desperately to shrink their bodies.

The psychological phenomenon of **body dysmorphia** is prevalent. Even when a patient manages the condition well, the trauma of living in a body that feels "out of control" can linger.

3. Social Stigma

Society judges weight harshly. Lipedema patients face bias in the workplace, in social settings, and even in healthcare. The assumption that the patient is "lazy" creates a barrier to empathy and effective treatment.

Validation is the First Step

Understanding the anatomy and physiology of Lipedema is not just an academic exercise; it is an act of validation.

- It validates that the pain is real, not imagined.
- It validates that the resistance to weight loss is physiological, not a lack of discipline.

- It validates that you are dealing with a chronic disease that requires medical management, not just a gym membership.

Now that we have defined the disorder and explored the biological mechanisms at play—the fibrosis, the inflammation, and the lymphatic strain—we can move forward. We are no longer fighting a mystery; we are managing a known entity. In the following chapters, we will use this biological understanding to construct a roadmap for treatment, covering everything from the physics of compression garments to the biochemistry of anti-inflammatory nutrition.

The foundation is laid. Let us now begin the work of reclaiming your health.

Chapter 2: Stages and Types of Lipedema

Lipedema is often described in clinical terms—stages, types, nodules, fat cuffs—but at its core it's a lived experience: for many people it begins as a strange mismatch between how their body looks and how it feels, and then slowly (or sometimes quickly) becomes a source of pain, bruising, limited mobility, and frustrating diagnostic confusion. In this chapter we'll walk through the commonly used stages and the classification of types, explain what's happening under the skin at each step, and highlight why distinguishing stages and types matters for diagnosis and care.

Why stages and types matter

Think of the staging system as a map and the type classification as a pin that shows where the condition is happening on the body. Staging helps clinicians and patients understand how far the disease has progressed whether it's largely cosmetic and early, or whether structural changes and complications are already present. The "type" of lipedema points to which areas are affected (hips, thighs, ankles, arms, calves), and that matters for mobility, clothing, compression strategies, and (if needed) surgical planning.

Those systems are not perfect; lipedema often overlaps with obesity, venous disease, or lymphedema, and people don't always fit neatly into a single box but they provide a shared language that improves diagnosis, aids research, and helps guide treatment choices. Authoritative clinical summaries and reviews describe the stages and types used in practice today.

The four stages — what clinicians look (and feel) for

Most clinicians and specialist centers use a three-stage morphological system (smooth → nodular → lobular), but many references and patient-facing sources also include a fourth stage that recognizes the development of combined lymphatic problems (lipolymphedema). Below is a practical, patient-centered description of each stage—what you might see, what you might feel, and what's happening biologically.

Stage 1 — early, smooth but abnormal fat

What it looks and feels like: the skin surface appears smooth and normal to the eye. Under the skin, however, the subcutaneous fat layer is thicker and often has a nodular feel — clinicians describe it as "peas under the skin" or a slightly grainy texture on palpation. Patients commonly report tenderness, heightened sensitivity to pressure, and easy bruising even at this stage.

What's happening biologically: the fat lobules (small packages of fat and connective tissue) enlarge and the extracellular matrix begins to change. There's early microvascular and connective tissue remodeling small blood vessels are fragile (hence bruising) and the lymphatic microcirculation may already be stressed. Early fibrosis (hardening of connective tissue) may be minimal but begins to develop beneath the smooth surface. These clinical features and the "pea-nodular" feel are described in clinical reviews and patient resources.

Why early recognition matters: because interventions that reduce pain and improve mobility (manual lymphatic drainage, compression, tailored exercise, symptom-focused nutrition counseling) can be started before major structural changes occur. Also, early diagnosis helps avoid the common mislabeling of lipedema as "simply obesity," which leads to frustrating and often ineffective weight-loss-only strategies.

Stage 2 — nodular, dimpled, and more symptomatic

What it looks and feels like: the skin surface becomes uneven — dimpling, indentations, and a "quilted" or "orange-peel" appearance may appear. The subcutaneous fat becomes more nodular and palpable. Larger fat lobules form and small lipomas or fibrotic nodules may be felt. Pain and tenderness often increase, and mobility can become more challenging as the fat deposit grows.

What's happening biologically: the fat tissue becomes more fibrotic and nodular, and connective tissue septa thicken, producing the visible change in skin texture. Microvascular fragility persists and inflammatory signaling in the adipose tissue increases. Clinically, this stage is important because the tissue is less likely to respond to conservative measures alone, and symptoms such as heaviness, aching, and sensitivity typically increase. Authoritative clinical summaries describe this transition from smooth to nodular fat as the hallmark of stage 2.

Practical implications: staged compression garments fitted by a trained clinician, combined decongestive therapies, and tailored physical therapy can reduce symptoms and slow progression. Patients often benefit from coaching on pacing, pain management, and joint-sparing exercise because the added weight and nodularity can change gait and joint loads.

Stage 3 — lobular, large deformations, mechanical impact

What it looks and feels like: large lobules and overhangs of fatty tissue develop, often around the outer and inner thighs, knees, and lower legs. The legs can take on a pronounced, bulky appearance; walking and daily movement may be noticeably impaired. Skin can fold and rub, increasing the risk of skin irritation and infection in skin folds.

What's happening biologically: long-standing adipose tissue expansion is accompanied by increased fibrosis, altered lymphatic and microvascular function, and more persistent inflammation. The fat deposits form large lobules that distort the limb shape and can create mechanical barriers to mobility. Many surgical reports and clinic guides describe stage 3 as the "lobular" stage where tissue architecture is significantly altered.

Treatment considerations: when stage 3 is present, conservative measures may still provide symptom relief (pain reduction, improved sleep, better mobility), but many patients consider specialized surgical options (lipedema-focused tumescent liposuction or water-assisted liposuction performed by surgeons experienced with lipedema tissue). Surgical planning must account for increased bleeding risk and potential lymphatic damage; outcomes often improve quality of life but are not a cure and require ongoing multidisciplinary care.

Stage 4 — lipolymphedema (combined lymphedema and lipedema)

What it looks and feels like: stage 4 refers to the coexistence of lipedema and clinically significant lymphedema. Patients have the disproportionate adipose deposits of lipedema plus the fluid-protein accumulation and pitting edema typical of lymphedema. There may be large overhanging folds of tissue, and the affected limbs can be heavy, prone to infections (cellulitis), and hard to move.

What's happening biologically: chronic adipose expansion and fibrosis have overwhelmed or damaged lymphatic drainage capacity, producing secondary lymphedema. Lymphatic collectors can become incompetent or compressed by the abnormal fat architecture, resulting in classical lymphedema features: pitting initially, then non-pitting, and skin/tissue changes. Clinical resources and specialty reviews recognize lipolymphedema as an advanced and important clinical state to identify.

Why identifying lipolymphedema is critical: because lymphedema requires specific management (complete decongestive therapy, careful skin care, possibly pneumatic compression, and specialized bandaging). If left unrecognized, treatments that ignore lymphatic dysfunction may be ineffective or even harmful.

How the stages were developed (brief history and limitations)

The three-stage morphological description appears in German surgical/clinical literature going back to early 2000s and has been adopted widely because it reflects visible and palpable tissue changes (smooth → nodular → lobular). Patient advocacy and specialty centers commonly add stage 4 to capture the frequent coexistence of lymphatic disease. These systems are descriptive rather than strictly pathophysiologic; they don't capture every variation or the pace at which an individual moves through stages. That said, they're useful for communication and research.

Types of lipedema — where the fat collects matters

Types of lipedema are defined by the anatomical distribution of abnormal subcutaneous fat. Clinically the types are labeled Type I through Type V (and occasionally mixed patterns are seen). Knowing the type shapes practical decisions: which garment shapes will fit, where to place compression, whether arm symptoms will limit function, and how to plan surgical approaches.

Below is a clinically useful breakdown of the types, with notes on how they commonly present and why each matters.

Type I — pelvis and buttocks (navel to hips)

Presentation: fat accumulates between the navel and hips, covering the pelvic region and buttocks. This is often an early presentation and can give a patient a disproportionate pelvis/hip profile compared with the upper body.

Clinical consequences: early gait and posture changes can develop if the pelvic/hip load is asymmetric. Clothing fit around the waist and hips becomes difficult; pain and tenderness in sitting or certain movements may occur.

Type II — pelvis to knees

Presentation: fat extends from the pelvis down to the knees. A typical sign is the formation of fat folds above the knees and disproportionate fullness of the thighs.

Clinical consequences: this pattern often begins to limit mobility sooner than Type I because bulk at the distal thigh and around the knees interferes with walking and climbing stairs.

Type III — pelvis to ankles (ankle cuff)

Presentation: fat accumulation runs from pelvis to ankle and is often accompanied by the classic "ankle cuff" — an abrupt stop of abnormal fat at the ankle, sparing the feet (or sparing the dorsum of the feet). This "cuff" is a hallmark often used clinically to separate lipedema from other causes of swelling.

Clinical consequences: severe difficulty with mobility; the visual and mechanical impact is large and often triggers patients to seek specialist care. This is one of the most functionally limiting types. The type system and the ankle-cuff description are widely used in clinical references.

Type IV — arms (shoulders to wrists)

Presentation: abnormal fat deposition affects the arms from the shoulders to the wrists. This can be unilateral or bilateral.

Clinical consequences: patients report heaviness, reduced range of motion, and discomfort with tasks like lifting, dressing, or reaching. Compression sleeves and careful physical therapy are often part of conservative management.

Type V — calves only (rare)

Presentation: predominantly in the calves, producing a column-like appearance of the lower legs. This presentation is less common but recognized in clinical images and reports.

Clinical consequences: localized pain and altered gait mechanics; because it's rare, it may be misdiagnosed as other localized adipose or vascular conditions unless a clinician is familiar with lipedema patterns.

Mixed patterns also occur: many patients don't fit perfectly into a single type and may have overlapping areas. Imaging (ultrasound) and careful examination help confirm distribution and rule out other causes.

Why lipedema fat behaves differently — a short primer

One of the most clinically important observations is that lipedema fat is not simply "extra weight" that will respond predictably to diet and exercise. While general weight loss can reduce overall body fat, the abnormal, symmetrically distributed lipedema fat tends to be resistant to conventional caloric-restriction approaches. Several clinical reviews and primary studies have documented this resistance and emphasize that lipedema is a distinct adipose tissue disorder with microvascular, connective tissue, and lymphatic involvement. These differences help explain why patients often feel frustrated by "lose weight" advice that does not help the painful, disproportionate limb fullness.

Emerging research links hormonal influences (notably estrogen pathways), genetic susceptibility, and local inflammatory and microvascular changes as drivers of the abnormal fat behavior. The common clinical pattern — onset or worsening during puberty, pregnancy, or menopause — supports the role of hormonal triggers. Recent systematic reviews and open-access articles review these mechanisms in detail.

Distinguishing lipedema from other conditions

Lipedema is commonly misattributed to obesity, lymphedema, or simple localized adiposity. Here are practical differentiators clinicians use:

- **Symmetry and distribution:** lipedema is typically bilateral and symmetric, often stopping at the ankles (ankle cuff) while sparing the feet; obesity is more proportional and generalized.
- **Pain and easy bruising:** lipedema tissue is tender and bruises easily; simple obesity usually isn't painful in the subcutaneous tissue itself.
- **Response to diet/exercise:** lipedema adipose is comparatively resistant to weight loss through diet and exercise.
- **Pitting:** lymphedema shows pitting edema (especially early on) and may be unilateral or asymmetric; lipedema alone usually does not show significant pitting unless lymphedema develops.
- **Stemmer sign:** a clinical test often used for lymphedema (ability to pinch the skin on the dorsum of the toes/fingers); its absence helps suggest lipedema, though it's not infallible.

Comprehensive reviews contrast these disorders and emphasize the need for combined clinical, imaging, and sometimes lymphoscintigraphy assessments when the diagnosis is uncertain.

Clinical implications of stage and type for treatment planning

Understanding where a patient sits in the staging/type framework allows clinicians and patients to choose realistic, staged interventions:

1. **Conservative, symptom-directed care (early → all stages):**
    - Manual lymphatic drainage and decongestive therapy when there are lymphatic symptoms.
    - Fitted compression garments (different profiles for thighs vs. calves vs. arms).
    - Pain management strategies, skin care, and infection prevention.
    - Joint-sparing exercise (water therapy, low-impact strength training).
    - Nutritional counseling focused on symptom control and metabolic health rather than unrealistic promises of reversing lipedema fat.
    Evidence reviews note there is no diet proven to cure lipedema, though individualized nutrition can reduce symptoms and improve overall health.

2. **Advanced supportive care (stage 2–3):**
    - Focus on mobility aids if necessary, targeted physical therapy, and optimization of skin health.
    - Psychological and social support — body image, chronic pain, and mobility limitations all carry emotional load.

2. **Surgical options (most commonly considered in stage 2–3, sometimes stage 4):**
    - Specialized liposuction techniques aimed at removing pathological adipose tissue can reduce pain and improve

function for many patients. These are not cosmetic procedures in the lipedema context: they can be therapeutic, but require surgeons experienced in lipedema and careful post-op care (compression, lymphatic-preserving technique). Surgery does not guarantee permanent prevention of recurrence and must be paired with lifelong conservative care. Surgical literature also stresses the need to protect and preserve lymphatic channels to avoid causing or worsening lymphedema.

3. **When lymphedema is present (stage 4 / lipolymphedema):**
    - Standard lymphedema care (complete decongestive therapy, bandaging, careful skin surveillance) becomes central. Collaboration between lymphedema specialists and lipedema-experienced surgeons is ideal.

A note on research, uncertainty, and emerging perspectives

Although knowledge about lipedema has increased substantially over the last decade, there remain uncertainties: the precise molecular triggers, the best non-surgical disease-modifying therapies, and standardized outcome measures for surgical success are still active research areas. Recent systematic reviews and clinical overviews emphasize the hormonal and genetic hypotheses and call for better diagnostic biomarkers and randomized controlled trials of interventions. For patients, this means that management is often individualized, and multidisciplinary care (specialist physicians, physiotherapists, lymphedema therapists, and surgeons familiar with lipedema) offers the best outcomes.

Practical guidance — questions to ask your clinician (and what to expect)

If you or someone you care for is being evaluated for lipedema, these questions can make the visit more productive:

- Where do you think I fall in the staging system, and what features led you to that conclusion?
- What type (I–V) best describes my pattern of fat distribution?
- Are there signs my lymphatic system is involved (lipolymphedema)?
- What conservative measures do you recommend right now (compression, MLD, exercise plans)?
- Do you think I'm a candidate for surgical treatment now or in the future, and what would that involve?
- What outcomes should I realistically expect from conservative care and, separately, from surgery?

A good clinician will use staging and local distribution to guide a tailored plan, and will be frank about what conservative measures can accomplish versus when surgical referral might be reasonable.

Stages and types are more than academic labels — they are practical tools that connect a patient's symptoms, function, and goals with appropriate care. Early recognition and a compassionate, evidence-informed approach reduce pain, preserve function, and improve quality of life. If you suspect lipedema, ask for a careful clinical evaluation by a clinician experienced in fat disorders or a lymphedema/lipedema center. The right diagnosis is the first step toward the right combination of care for the long run.

Chapter 3 — Causes and Risk Factors of Lipedema

Lipedema often feels like a riddle: excess, painful fat that appears in predictable patterns, mainly in women, sometimes runs in families, and commonly flares during life's hormonal milestones. Yet despite decades of clinical observation and growing research, the exact cause remains incompletely understood. This chapter walks through the strongest clues researchers and clinicians have gathered so far — genetics, hormones, body composition, inflammation, and environment — and explains what each means for someone living with or at risk for lipedema.

A quick orientation: why causes matter

Knowing the drivers of lipedema matters for patients and clinicians because it shapes expectations and choices. If lipedema were simply "bad lifestyle choices," the clinical message would be straightforward (eat less, move more). But evidence shows the reality is much more complex: lipedema is a distinct disorder of subcutaneous fat with vascular, connective-tissue, and lymphatic elements. That complexity explains why purely weight-focused approaches often fail to address the pain, bruising, and disproportion seen in lipedema. For authoritative clinical overviews that summarize these differences, see resources such as NCBI Bookshelf and Cleveland Clinic.

Genetic predisposition — the family clue

One of the strongest signals that lipedema is at least partly inherited is its tendency to cluster in families. Multiple studies report that a substantial fraction of patients have a first-degree relative with a similar fat distribution or documented lipedema. Large family-based analyses and clinical series support a heritable component, with patterns consistent with autosomal dominant transmission and incomplete penetrance in many pedigrees.

What that means in practice:

- If your mother, grandmother, or sister has predictable, painful fat deposits on the legs or arms, your risk is higher than someone without that family history.
- Genetic research so far suggests *heterogeneity* — not one single "lipedema gene" but multiple genetic contributors that interact with other factors. Recent family studies have moved the field away from a single-gene explanation and toward a model where several variants (some common, some rare) change susceptibility.

Why this matters for patients: genetic predisposition helps explain why lipedema develops despite efforts at weight control and why it runs in families, and it also directs research toward identifying biomarkers that might one day help with earlier diagnosis or targeted therapies.

Hormonal influences — the timing clue

Lipedema nearly always affects women and typically begins or worsens during periods of hormonal change: puberty, pregnancy, and menopause are classic trigger windows. That temporal pattern points strongly to sex hormones — especially estrogen — playing a central role. Reviews and mechanistic studies link estrogen signaling to differences in subcutaneous adipose tissue distribution and behavior, and several clinical reviews recast lipedema as a hormonally influenced disorder distinct from generalized obesity.

Clinical features that line up with hormonal influence:

- **Onset at puberty:** many women (and older girls) report the first notable leg fullness or tenderness after puberty.
- **Pregnancy and postpartum changes:** pregnancy frequently accelerates visible fat accumulation or symptom severity.
- **Perimenopause and menopause:** hormonal shifts again correlate with progression in some patients.

Mechanisms under research include:

- Estrogen receptor differences in subcutaneous fat cells that might favor fat expansion in specific body regions.
- Interactions between sex steroids and local microvascular or lymphatic function, leading to increased capillary fragility and tissue fluid changes.
- Hormone-driven differences in fat-cell progenitors and the extracellular matrix that could favor the abnormal fat pattern in lipedema.

In short: the "when" of lipedema onset gives us a powerful clue that hormones matter — and that treatments or prevention strategies that ignore hormonal biology may miss an important piece of the disease puzzle.

Body composition and obesity — an important but distinct relationship

Obesity and lipedema are often conflated, but the relationship is nuanced. Larger body mass index (BMI) is common among people with lipedema, and excess weight can worsen symptoms (mechanical strain, joint pain, reduced mobility), but obesity is not a necessary or sufficient cause. In other words, lipedema can exist in people of normal weight, and being overweight does not explain the characteristic symmetric, painful fat distribution that defines lipedema. Clinical resources note that many patients with lipedema have elevated BMI values, and some clinics report a substantial proportion with BMI > 35, but interpretation of those numbers requires care because BMI poorly captures the distinctive, gynoid fat pattern seen in lipedema.

Key takeaways:

- Excess weight amplifies symptoms: carrying more mass increases joint stress and may magnify mobility problems and discomfort.
- Weight loss affects central/visceral fat more than lipedema fat: many patients notice global weight loss but little change in the disproportionate lower-body fat.
- Alternative measures (waist-to-height ratio, body composition scans) sometimes give a different picture than BMI and may better reflect metabolic risk in this population. Studies suggest BMI alone can overstate "obesity" prevalence in lipedema cohorts, because the condition preferentially deposits subcutaneous fat in the lower body rather than centrally.

Clinical implication: weight management is still part of supportive care (for cardiovascular and functional reasons) but it must be paired with other, lipedema-targeted strategies (compression, lymphatic care, specialized physical therapy, and, when appropriate, liposuction techniques designed for lipedema tissue).

Inflammation, microvascular changes, and extracellular matrix — the tissue-level clues

Lipedema fat behaves differently at the tissue level. Compared to normal adipose or obesity-related adipose, lipedema tissue shows changes in microvessels, immune cell infiltration, and connective tissue architecture. Several histological and imaging studies have demonstrated:

- Increased microvascular fragility and capillary permeability (which contributes to easy bruising).
- Local inflammatory signaling and immune cell presence in the fat.
- Fibrosis or thickening of connective-tissue septa that organize fat lobules, leading to the nodular and lobular textures clinicians feel on exam.

These features explain common symptoms: pain, easy bruising, sensitivity to pressure, and a tendency for tissue to feel "thicker" or more nodular. The inflammation is not necessarily the same as the systemic inflammatory state seen in metabolically unhealthy obesity; instead, many studies suggest lipedema represents a localized adipose-tissue disorder with distinct immune and extracellular-matrix activity.

Practical clinical notes:

- Treating inflammation and supporting microvascular health (through compression, gentle decongestive care, and inflammation-aware lifestyle changes) can reduce symptoms even if the underlying fat remains.
- Anti-inflammatory diets or metabolic interventions may help symptom burden for some patients, but they are not a cure for lipedema fat itself. Research continues into whether targeted anti-inflammatory or anti-fibrotic therapies could change disease progression.

Lymphatic involvement and the risk of lipolymphedema

Lipedema and lymphedema are distinct but interrelated. In many cases, prolonged lipedema-related tissue change eventually overwhelms lymphatic drainage or physically disrupts collectors, producing a secondary lymphedema component — often called lipolymphedema. When lymphatic dysfunction appears, patients gain additional swelling, pitting may develop, and the management priorities shift to include lymphedema-focused care (complete decongestive therapy, meticulous skin care, and bandaging). Recognizing lymphatic involvement early is important because it changes both conservative and surgical planning. Clinical reviews and specialty centers highlight this progression and the need for multidisciplinary management when lymphatic signs are present.

Lifestyle and environmental influences — triggers and amplifiers

Lifestyle factors don't cause lipedema in the genetic-and-hormonal sense, but they can amplify symptoms, influence progression speed, and determine overall health outcomes. Sedentary behavior, poor cardiorespiratory fitness, chronic stress, and diets that promote systemic inflammation are common amplifiers. Environmental and behavioral factors interact with the underlying susceptibility to shape how quickly and how severely the condition becomes symptomatic.

Clinical guidance often recommends:

- Regular, joint-sparing physical activity (walking, water-based exercise, controlled strengthening) to support mobility and lymphatic flow.
- Compression garments to support tissues and reduce discomfort during activity.
- Attention to sleep, stress reduction, and anti-inflammatory dietary patterns as supportive measures — useful for symptom control and general health but unlikely by themselves to reverse lipedema fat.

Case vignette (illustrative): a woman with a family history of lipedema notices increased leg tenderness and fullness after a busy pregnancy; she becomes less active because of musculoskeletal pain, gains weight, and within a year reports more pronounced nodularity. This common pattern illustrates how hormonal triggers, genetic background, and lifestyle interact.

Coexisting medical conditions that can influence risk or presentation

Several conditions frequently appear alongside lipedema and can complicate diagnosis or management:

- **Venous disease:** chronic venous insufficiency can cause leg swelling and skin changes that overlap with lipedema signs. Differentiation is important because treatments differ.
- **Metabolic disorders:** while lipedema fat is less metabolically active than visceral fat, many patients have metabolic comorbidities (e.g., insulin resistance, dyslipidemia) or obesity that require attention. Recent studies report a mixed metabolic profile and emphasize individualized assessment.
- **Autoimmune or inflammatory disorders:** chronic inflammation from other sources can compound pain and swelling; clinicians frequently take a broad view of inflammatory contributors when evaluating symptoms.

How risk factors inform prevention and early action (realistic expectations)

We do not yet have proven strategies that reliably prevent lipedema in someone with genetic susceptibility. However, knowledge of risk factors helps with early recognition and reasonable, targeted interventions:

- If you have a strong family history, watch for early signs during puberty, pregnancy, or major hormonal transitions and seek evaluation if pain, symmetric leg fullness, or easy bruising appear. Early conservative care can reduce symptoms and preserve mobility.
- Address modifiable amplifiers: maintain cardiovascular fitness, manage weight for overall health (even though lipedema fat is resistant to diet-only approaches), reduce inflammatory behaviors (smoking, poor sleep), and manage stress. These steps don't "cure" lipedema but improve quality of life and reduce secondary harms.

Research frontiers — what scientists are testing next

The field is actively exploring:

- **Genetics:** large family and population studies to identify risk variants and better define inheritance patterns. Recent family-based exome studies point toward genetic heterogeneity rather than a single causative gene.
- **Hormone-adipose interactions:** more detailed work on estrogen receptor signaling in affected fat and how this changes fat-lobule biology during life stages.
- **Immunology and fibrosis:** clarifying the exact immune cells and signaling pathways that drive local inflammation and connective-tissue remodeling, with an eye toward targeted anti-inflammatory or anti-fibrotic drugs.
- **Better diagnostics and biomarkers:** objective tests that distinguish lipedema from obesity, lymphedema, and venous disease — which would speed diagnosis and allow earlier, more tailored therapy.

Practical questions to bring to a clinician

If you suspect lipedema or have risk factors, these questions focus the visit and help produce a plan:

- Do I have features consistent with lipedema or another cause of lower-body swelling?
- Is there evidence of lymphatic involvement? What tests would you recommend?

- How does my family history inform prognosis and treatment choices?
- What conservative measures would you prioritize now (compression, manual drainage, exercise)?
- Am I a candidate for surgical referral? If so, what outcomes should I expect and what are the risks?

Final thoughts — complexity, compassion, and partnership

Lipedema is a multifactorial disorder where inherited susceptibility, hormonal milieu, tissue-level changes, and lifestyle/environmental factors intersect. For patients, this means the path forward is rarely a single treatment or a single "cause" to eliminate. The best outcomes come from a partnership: careful diagnosis, symptom-directed conservative care started early, attention to overall health, and access to specialists when needed. Research is advancing — genetics, hormone biology, and tissue immunology are promising avenues — but right now, clinicians can offer validated symptom management and surgical options for selected patients, and a growing community of specialists and researchers is working to translate scientific insights into better prevention and treatment.

Chapter 4 — Lipedema vs. Other Conditions

When I first learned about lipedema, I remember thinking: "So is it swollen legs? Is it obesity? Is it just cellulite?" That confusion is exactly what people face in clinic rooms every day — patients who've been told to "lose weight," or those who've been referred down the wrong diagnostic pathway because the differences between similar conditions look subtle at first glance. This chapter walks you through the key distinctions between lipedema and the conditions it's most often confused with: lymphedema, obesity, cellulite, and lipodystrophy — and also touches on venous disease and mixed presentations. My aim is practical: give you clear signs to notice, what tests clinicians use, and how these differences change treatment and expectations.

Why does accurate differentiation matter ?

Imagine two people who both have heavy, tender legs. One has lipedema; the other has lymphedema from cancer surgery. The treatments, prognosis, and daily management are not the same. Misdiagnosis can delay helpful therapies, leave people with unnecessary blame, and even lead to harmful interventions. Clear differentiation helps patients get the right combination of conservative care, surgical options when appropriate, lymphatic therapy, or metabolic support.

Below I'll break down each comparison into (1) what it looks and feels like clinically, (2) simple bedside tests and clues, and (3) what the diagnosis means for treatment and expectations.

Lipedema vs. Lymphedema

What they are, in plain terms

- **Lipedema** is a chronic disorder of subcutaneous fat distribution that typically affects both legs symmetrically (and sometimes the arms), causes pain and easy bruising, and tends to spare the feet.
- **Lymphedema** is swelling caused by impaired lymphatic drainage — fluid (and later protein-rich tissue changes) accumulates, producing puffiness that often includes the feet and can be asymmetric.

These are different processes: one is primarily an abnormal expansion of fat with connective-tissue changes; the other is failure of the lymphatic drainage system leading to fluid accumulation and secondary tissue changes. Large clinical reviews that compare the two highlight both shared features (heaviness, limb enlargement, fibrosis over time) and crucial differences in distribution and physical exam.

Key bedside clues

- **Symmetry and distribution:** lipedema is classically bilateral and symmetric; lymphedema can be unilateral or asymmetric and commonly involves the feet.
- **Pain and bruising:** spontaneous tenderness and easy bruising are hallmarks of lipedema; lymphedema is typically not

painful from palpation in the early fluid-only stages (pain arises later from chronic tissue changes or infection).

- **Stemmer sign:** inability to pinch the skin at the base of the toes (a positive Stemmer sign) suggests lymphedema; it is usually absent in isolated lipedema.
- **Pitting:** early lymphedema often shows pitting on pressure; lipedema typically does not pit unless lymphatic failure develops (lipolymphedema).
- **Onset and triggers:** lipedema often begins at hormonal milestones (puberty, pregnancy, menopause); lymphedema often follows lymphatic injury (surgery, radiation) or is congenital.

Why it matters for treatment

If lymphatic dysfunction is present (true lymphedema or lipolymphedema), therapies such as complete decongestive therapy (manual lymphatic drainage, bandaging, skin care) and careful monitoring for infections (cellulitis) are essential. If symptoms are driven mainly by lipedema tissue without lymphatic failure, compression, pain management, and (in selected cases) specialized liposuction techniques aimed at removing pathological fat are considered. Because these distinctions change the therapeutic pathway, accurate assessment early can change outcomes.

Lipedema vs. Obesity

The important conceptual difference

Obesity is an excess of body fat that is generally distributed according to a person's overall energy balance and genetics. Lipedema is a particular pattern of abnormal, painful fat deposition in the limbs that is resistant to dieting in the areas affected. While the two conditions can co-exist, and many people with lipedema have higher BMI, conflating them leads to dismissive advice ("if you just lose weight this will go away") that is often wrong and harmful.

Clinical guides and patient resources emphasize that lipedema fat shows different behavior (pain, bruising, resistance to typical weight loss) and a different distribution (disproportionate lower-body fat, sparing the trunk) compared with generalized obesity. This difference is central to why management strategies need to be tailored.

Practical differentiators clinicians use

- **Distribution:** lipedema typically produces a gynoid pattern — hips, outer and inner thighs, often down to the ankle with an "ankle cuff," sometimes affecting arms. Obesity is more generalized, and central (abdominal) fat is common.
- **Response to weight loss:** with calorie restriction and exercise, overall body weight may fall but the disproportionate limb fat of lipedema often remains. Patients frequently report losing weight from the trunk while the legs remain stubbornly large.
- **Tenderness and bruising:** pain with pressure and easy bruising strongly suggest lipedema rather than obesity alone.
- **Metabolic profile:** obesity often associates with metabolic syndrome markers (insulin resistance, dyslipidemia), whereas lipedema fat itself appears to have a different metabolic signature; however, many patients have both lipedema and metabolic risk factors, so assessment is individualized.

Treatment implications

Weight management remains important for cardiovascular and joint health, but it is not a specific cure for lipedema. Conservative lipedema care (compression, manual lymphatic techniques, exercise, and targeted skin/joint care) should be provided alongside broader lifestyle measures. When surgical removal of lipedema tissue is considered, it is not primarily cosmetic — many patients report meaningful symptom relief after lipedema-focused liposuction.

Lipedema vs. Cellulite

Why they get confused

Visually, both lipedema and cellulite can produce lumpy, dimpled skin in the thighs and buttocks. But the similarity largely ends at appearance: cellulite is a common, benign cosmetic change in the dermis and subcutaneous fat architecture and is not typically painful or progressive in the way lipedema can be.

Authoritative patient-facing resources and expert clinicians stress that cellulite is cosmetic — not a disease — while lipedema is a medical, progressive condition that produces pain, bruising, and functional limitations for many. When in doubt, a clinician's evaluation for tenderness, symmetry, and progression helps separate the two.

Quick bedside distinctions

- **Pain:** cellulite is usually not tender; lipedema commonly is.
- **Progression:** cellulite is cosmetic and rarely progresses into the painful, nodular, limb-enlarging pattern of lipedema. Lipedema typically worsens over time without appropriate management.

- **Response to treatment:** cellulite may respond to cosmetic procedures and topical approaches; lipedema requires medical management and sometimes specialized surgical approaches for symptom relief.

Why the difference matters

Labeling lipedema as "cellulite" delays effective care and can invalidate a patient's pain. Educating clinicians and patients about these distinctions shortens the path to appropriate therapies.

Lipedema vs. Lipodystrophy

What lipodystrophy is

Lipodystrophy describes conditions where fat is lost from certain parts of the body (localized or generalized), often with metabolic consequences. It's essentially the opposite pattern from lipedema: loss of fat rather than painful, abnormal accumulation. Lipodystrophies can be genetic (congenital) or acquired (for example, in people on certain medications).

Scientific comparative analyses highlight that the molecular signatures of lipedema and lipodystrophy differ — both at the level of gene expression and tissue histology — which supports treating the two as distinct entities. Clinicians use that difference to guide metabolic evaluation and management: lipodystrophy often requires aggressive metabolic treatment and monitoring, whereas lipedema management prioritizes symptom control, lymphatic care, and body-shape functional strategies.

Why people mix them up

To a non-expert, "weird fat" in a limb may look like either more fat or less fat depending on where you start, and body-shape changes in both groups can be dramatic. But the clinical story (painful enlargement vs. loss of tissue and metabolic disturbance) usually clarifies the diagnosis.

Other conditions that commonly enter the differential

Chronic venous insufficiency (CVI)

CVI causes edema, skin discoloration, and sometimes lipodermatosclerosis (skin and subcutaneous tissue changes) that can mimic or coexist with lipedema. A helpful difference: venous disease often causes relatively more dependent swelling (worse at the end of the day), visible varicose veins, and skin changes localized to areas drained by incompetent veins. Duplex ultrasound of the veins is the go-to test for venous disease.

Lipohypertrophy and mixed pictures

There are patients whose presentations overlap — for example, lipedema with venous insufficiency, or lipedema with secondary lymphatic compromise (lipolymphedema). These mixed pictures are common and are why a detailed history, physical exam, and sometimes imaging are essential.

Tests and tools clinicians use to tell them apart

No single test gives a definitive answer every time. Thoughtful diagnosis usually combines history, careful physical exam, and selective imaging.

History & physical exam (first-line)

- Onset timing (puberty/pregnancy/menopause vs. surgery/injury)
- Symmetry and distribution (ankle cuff, foot sparing)
- Pain and bruising
- Stemmer sign, pitting, and skin texture (nodular vs. spongy)
These remain the most powerful differentiators at the bedside — experienced clinicians can often make an accurate clinical diagnosis from history and exam alone. Several clinical reviews stress the importance of detailed palpation and distribution assessment.

Imaging

- **Ultrasound:** increasingly used to examine subcutaneous tissue architecture, vascularity, and to rule out other causes (venous or localized masses).
- **Lymphoscintigraphy:** nuclear medicine studies that track lymph flow are helpful when lymphedema is suspected or to confirm lymphatic dysfunction.
- **MRI/CT:** rarely required for straightforward cases, but helpful if other structural problems are suspected.

Lab and metabolic testing

There is no blood test that diagnoses lipedema, but clinicians often screen for metabolic comorbidities (lipid panels, glucose, thyroid function) and inflammatory markers where appropriate.

Common diagnostic pitfalls and how to avoid them

1. **"It's just obesity"** — A frequent, harmful reflex. Ask whether the disproportion is painful, symmetric, and resistant to prior weight loss efforts. If so, investigate lipedema.
2. **"It's just cellulite"** — Cellulite is common and not painful; if there is tenderness, progression, or functional decline, consider lipedema.
3. **Overlooking mixed disease** — Don't assume a single cause when the picture is complex; venous disease, lipedema, and lymphedema often coexist and require combined approaches.
4. **Failing to recognize lymphatic involvement** — If swelling includes the feet, if there is pitting, or if infections occur, evaluate for lymphedema since the treatment priorities change.

A careful, compassionate clinician who listens to the history, examines distribution and tenderness, and uses imaging judiciously will usually avoid these pitfalls.

What the differences mean for patients — practical examples

- **If you have lipedema:** you can expect a focus on symptom control (compression, pain strategies, targeted exercise), prevention of lymphatic overload, and in some cases, referral for specialized liposuction techniques that remove pathological fat and decrease pain. Realistic expectation-setting is important: treatment reduces symptoms and improves function and quality of life, but lipedema is typically a chronic condition that needs ongoing management.

- **If you have lymphedema:** your immediate priorities are lymphatic drainage, infection prevention, and preserving limb function with compression and bandaging; surgical strategies differ and are often targeted to improve lymphatic flow or remove fluid-rich tissue.
- **If you have obesity with no lipedema:** metabolic health, weight management, and exercise will be the main focus, and expectations about where fat will reduce should be discussed honestly.
- **If you have a mixed picture:** coordinated multidisciplinary care (vascular, lymphatic, obesity, physical therapy, and sometimes surgical specialists) produces the best outcomes.

Questions to bring to your clinician (short checklist)

- Based on my history and exam, what condition(s) are you most concerned about?
- Are my feet involved, and what does that indicate?
- Was the Stemmer sign performed? What was the result?
- Would imaging (ultrasound or lymphoscintigraphy) change management?
- Which conservative measures should I start immediately?
- Am I a candidate for surgery, and what are the expected benefits and risks?

Asking specific, practical questions like these changes visits from vague reassurance to targeted planning.

Final thoughts — diagnosis is the first treatment

Differentiating lipedema from lymphedema, obesity, cellulite, and lipodystrophy is not academic hair-splitting — it's the foundation of good care. The clinician's job is detective work: gather the history, look closely at distribution and signs, use targeted tests, and then explain clearly to the person in front of them what the diagnosis means for daily life and for realistic treatment goals. For patients, knowing the distinctions helps cut through the frustration of "try this diet" or "it's just cosmetic," and opens the door to meaningful symptom relief and improved function.

Part II: Non-Surgical Management

Chapter 5 — The Role of Compression Therapy

If lipedema has a daily "toolbox," compression therapy is one of the tools people reach for first. It's practical, non-invasive, and—when fitted and used correctly—can ease pain, reduce swelling, support mobility, and make life a little more manageable. This chapter explains, in a straightforward and human way, how compression works, what types of garments and devices are available, the evidence behind their use, how to choose and wear them, common problems and solutions, and when to combine compression with other treatments. I'll keep the science accessible and point to the best evidence so you — or a clinician you bring this chapter to — can make sensible, realistic decisions.

Why compression matters for people with lipedema

Compression therapy does three practical things for many people with lipedema:

1. **Reduces subjective symptoms** — pain, heaviness, tightness and tenderness often improve while garments are worn.
2. **Helps control fluid and microcirculatory leakage** — compression supports venous return and may reduce interstitial fluid that contributes to swelling and discomfort.

3. **Supports movement and skin integrity** — by stabilizing soft tissue and reducing friction and chafing, compression can make walking and exercise easier.

Put plainly: compression isn't a cure for the abnormal fat of lipedema, but it's a powerful symptom-management strategy that can reduce day-to-day suffering and improve function. Multiple clinical reviews and patient-care guidelines recommend compression as a core part of conservative care for lipedema and for cases with lymphatic involvement.

How compression works — the simple physiology

The physics behind compression therapy is intuitive: externally applied pressure reduces the diameter of superficial veins, helps propel blood and lymph centrally, and increases interstitial pressure so fluid is less likely to accumulate in the tissue. In lipedema, where capillary fragility and microvascular leakage may be present, that external support decreases the burden of excess interstitial fluid, reduces pain from tissue distension, and improves tissue comfort during activity. Pneumatic or intermittent devices add an active pumping element that mimics or amplifies natural muscle-pump action, which can be especially helpful after prolonged sitting or during rehabilitation. Clinical studies and reviews show measurable short-term improvements in leg circumference, bioimpedance (fluid markers), and patient-reported pain and tightness when compression is used, sometimes together with pneumatic compression.

Types of compression and when to use them

There's no single "best" garment for everyone with lipedema; the right choice depends on stage, limb shape, symptoms, comfort, and lifestyle. Below are the main options and practical strengths and limits of each.

1. Flat-knit compression garments

- **What they are:** Sturdier, less elastic garments knitted on flat machines; they provide firm, targeted pressure and are better for irregular limb shapes or larger limb volumes.
- **When to use:** Often recommended for stage 2 and stage 3 lipedema or when there are significant tissue nodularity and fibrosis. Clinical guidelines and specialist centers often favor flat-knit garments for their supportive profile.

2. Round-knit compression garments

- **What they are:** More elastic and seamless; comfortable for everyday wear and often easier to don.
- **When to use:** Good in early stages or for daytime comfort when robust shaping isn't needed; they are more forgiving with fit but offer less rigid support for lobular or very irregular tissue.

3. Compression sleeves (arms) and stockings (legs)

- **What they are:** Limb-specific garments in a range of compression classes and lengths.
- **When to use:** For localized arm or leg involvement. Sleeves can be layered with gauntlets or gloves when hand/forearm issues arise.

4. Adjustable wraps and Velcro systems

- **What they are:** Wraps that can be tightened or loosened throughout the day.
- **When to use:** For fluctuating edema, irregular limb shapes, or when donning is difficult. They're great for early morning swelling control or when you need variable compression.

5. Short-stretch bandaging and multilayer bandaging

- **What they are:** Bandages used in decongestive therapy; short-stretch is low-elasticity and works with muscle activity to pump fluid.
- **When to use:** Typically used in intensive therapy phases (for example, after a manual lymphatic drainage session) or when garments can't be fitted.

6. Pneumatic compression devices (PCDs)

- **What they are:** Electrically powered sleeves that rhythmically inflate and deflate to mimic lymphatic pumping.
- **When to use:** When at-home adjuncts are needed, after surgery, or in people who get greater relief from active sequential compression. Evidence suggests PCDs can reduce leg circumference and improve symptoms in lipedema, with measurable effect even after single sessions.

What the evidence says — realistic expectations

Compression therapy has solid support for symptom relief but limitations must be acknowledged clearly:

- **Symptom relief:** Multiple studies and clinical series show that compression reduces pain, tightness, and leg circumference measures and improves patient-reported outcomes (fatigue, function). Pneumatic devices show particularly strong short-term benefits.

- **Not a cure for lipedema fat:** Compression does not reliably remove lipedema adipose tissue or prevent disease progression on its own; it addresses fluid balance and pain rather than the pathological fat itself. Clinical consensus documents are explicit about compression being part of conservative management rather than a curative intervention.
- **Best when combined:** Studies comparing compression + exercise or compression + manual lymphatic drainage generally show better results than one intervention alone. Recent trials and observational work support combined approaches and highlight that individualized plans are key.

A balanced take: if you wear the right garment, fitted properly, you can expect meaningful symptom reduction that improves daily life. If you expect compression to "shrink" lipedema fat permanently, you're setting yourself up for disappointment. The best outcomes come from combining compression with other supportive measures and, where appropriate, surgical options for tissue removal.

Fitting: the difference between helpful and harmful

A garment that fits badly can be worse than none. Proper fitting matters for effectiveness, comfort, skin health, and compliance.

- **Get professionally fitted** whenever possible. Certified fitters (often through lymphedema or vascular clinics, or specialty suppliers) measure multiple points across the limb to select the correct pattern and compression class.

- **Compression class:** Medical/compression classes are expressed in mmHg (e.g., class 1, 2, 3). Higher classes give more pressure but may be harder to don and tolerate; your clinician should match class to your needs and stage.
- **Consider shape, not just size:** People with lipedema often have thigh/ankle disparities, bulky knees, or ankle cuffs that require special patterns (e.g., pantyhose vs. thigh highs, open-toe vs. closed). Flat-knit custom garments are often the best option for lumpy, irregular limbs.
- **Trial period:** Expect an adaptation period; garments should feel snug but not painfully tight. If you see skin blanching, numbness, increasing pain, or marks that do not resolve after removing the garment, stop and consult your fitter or clinician.

How long and how often should garments be worn?

Wear time is individualized, but common practical rules are:

- **Daily daytime use** is recommended for symptomatic relief—many people wear garments during waking hours and remove them at night.
- **During activity:** wearing compression during exercise or long periods of standing/walking delivers the most benefit for edema control and comfort.
- **After surgery or intensive decongestive therapy:** clinicians often recommend continuous compression (day and night) or specific protocols for a defined post-op period. Follow your surgical team's instructions.

Consistency is the key to benefit: sporadic use tends to produce sporadic results.

Combining compression with other therapies

Compression works best as one part of a multi-modal plan.

- **Manual Lymphatic Drainage (MLD):** gentle manual therapy followed by compression enhances fluid mobilization and patient comfort. While MLD alone has limited proven benefit for lipedema, added to compression it can improve outcomes in those with lymphatic involvement.
- **Exercise:** joint-sparing, muscle-activating exercises (water therapy, walking, resistance training) amplify compression benefits by using the muscle pump to move fluid centrally.
- **Weight and metabolic care:** keeping overall weight in a healthy range protects joints and cardiovascular health even if lipedema fat is resistant to diet alone.
- **Surgery:** if liposuction or lipedema reduction surgery is performed, compression is critical in the immediate post-op and maintenance phase to control swelling, support wounds, and optimize contour. PCDs and early mobilization are often part of the perioperative plan.

Troubleshooting common problems

Compression is immensely helpful, but it isn't always easy. Here are typical problems and practical fixes.

1. Moisture and skin irritation

- **Why it happens:** tight garments reduce airflow and can trap sweat.

- **Fixes:** use breathable, moisture-wicking liners; change garments daily; treat fungal or maceration issues promptly; consider cotton liners between garment and skin. Proper laundering and rotating multiple garments helps.

2. Donning and doffing is hard

- **Why it happens:** higher compression and tight seams make application difficult.
- **Fixes:** use donning aids (rubber gloves to improve grip, donning frames), consider zippered or Velcro-assisted garments, or adjustable wraps. Occupational therapists can teach techniques. Some suppliers offer lower-compression "training" garments for ease.

3. Pressure points and redness

- **Why it happens:** poor fit or seams hitting bony prominences.
- **Fixes:** get a refit; pad pressure points; ensure measurements were taken correctly and consider custom flat-knit options.

4. Allergic reactions or skin sensitivity

- **Why it happens:** materials like latex or certain dyes.
- **Fixes:** choose hypoallergenic fabrics; ask suppliers for composition; consider short-term topical treatments under clinician guidance.

5. Appearance and self-consciousness

- **Why it happens:** garments can be visible or change clothing fit.

- **Fixes:** modern medical garments come in a range of colors and styles; some suppliers offer custom cosmetic covers; counseling and peer support can help with body image concerns.

Special considerations

Pregnancy

Compression can be used during pregnancy to control swelling and discomfort, but fitting must be pregnancy-aware and supervised by a clinician. Consider maternity-specific garments and follow guidance on pressure classes.

Large limb volumes and custom garments

When off-the-shelf garments don't fit, custom, made-to-measure flat-knit garments are often the answer. They are more expensive but provide the correct pressure profile and dramatically improve comfort and effectiveness.

Access and cost

Compression can be expensive and insurance coverage varies widely. Work with suppliers and clinicians to explore coverage codes, custom garment funding options, and staged purchases (starting with day garments, then adding second garments for rotation).

When compression may not be enough (and what comes next)

For many people compression brings meaningful relief. For others—especially those with stage 2–3 disease and mechanical impairment—compression won't restore limb shape or fully control symptoms. In these cases, patients and clinicians often consider surgical options (lipedema-focused liposuction) alongside life-long conservative care. Importantly, compression continues to play a role after surgery to manage swelling and promote healing. Evidence and consensus documents recommend a combined, multidisciplinary strategy for best outcomes.

Practical checklist — what to ask at your first fitting

- What compression class do you recommend for my stage and symptoms?
- Do you offer flat-knit (custom) options for my limb shape?
- Can I try a garment before I buy, or do you offer a return trial?
- Which donning aids do you recommend and how do I use them?
- How should I launder and rotate garments?
- How often should I replace garments? (Typically every 6–12 months with daily use, sooner if elasticity declines.)

Final thoughts — compression as partnership, not punishment

Compression therapy works best when it's part of a compassionate, individualized plan. A well-fitted garment can relieve pain, let you move with less fear of chafing or heaviness, and make other self-care possible. It requires patience—an adaptation period, attention to skin care, and sometimes investment in custom solutions—but for many people it's a cornerstone of improved day-to-day life.

Chapter 6 — Nutritional Strategies for Living Better with Lipedema

Lipedema and diet have a complicated relationship. For many people the first thing they hear is "lose weight" — as if lipedema were simply stubborn fat that will fold away if you eat less. That's incomplete and often hurtful advice. The reality is more nuanced: while overall metabolic health and body weight matter for joint load and cardiovascular risk, lipedema fat behaves differently from ordinary fat. Nutrition doesn't *cure* the abnormal fat, but smart, evidence-informed dietary choices can reduce inflammation, support lymphatic and vascular health, improve pain and energy, and help a person feel more in control. This chapter walks through the best current nutritional approaches, the supplements with the most promising data, cautions about interactions and unrealistic promises, and practical meal and shopping guidance you can use tomorrow.

How nutrition helps (what it can — and can't — do)

First, a realistic frame: nutrition is one pillar in a multidimensional plan. It can:

- Lower systemic and tissue inflammation (which often reduces pain and tenderness).

- Improve vascular and lymphatic health indirectly (by improving endothelial function and reducing fluid-promoting diets).
- Support weight control for overall health (even if the disproportionate limb fat remains).
- Reduce comorbid metabolic risk (insulin resistance, dyslipidemia) that can worsen quality of life.

Nutrition alone is unlikely to remove lipedema fat or reverse structural tissue changes. But combined with compression, movement, lymphatic care, and—when needed—surgical options, targeted nutrition helps people feel better and can reduce symptom severity. Recent clinical overviews and review articles summarize these realistic, evidence-based benefits. NCBI Bookshelf.

The core dietary patterns that show promise

Several broad dietary patterns are commonly recommended for their anti-inflammatory, vascular-supporting, and metabolic benefits. Choice among them should be individualized to your preferences, cultural foodways, and medical needs.

1) Anti-inflammatory / Mediterranean-style eating (a gentle first-line choice)

What it looks like: plenty of vegetables and fruits, whole grains, legumes, nuts and seeds, extra-virgin olive oil, moderate fish and poultry, limited red meat, and minimal ultra-processed foods and added sugars.

Why it helps: this pattern is rich in polyphenols, fiber, and anti-inflammatory monounsaturated fats and omega-3s — all of which support vascular health and lower inflammatory markers. Several nutrition reviews and emerging lipedema studies highlight the benefits of Mediterranean-style elements for symptom burden and overall health. Nutrition Reviews. Practical note: it's sustainable for most people and supports broader cardiometabolic goals.

2) Lower-carbohydrate / ketogenic approaches (used in targeted trials)

What it looks like: a reduced carbohydrate intake with higher proportions of fat and moderate protein. Approaches range from low-carb (moderate restriction) to ketogenic (very low carb, high fat).

Why it helps: trials and recent controlled studies have reported improvements in pain and quality of life among women with lipedema following low-carbohydrate protocols. Mechanisms may include reduced systemic inflammation, changes in insulin signaling, and altered tissue metabolism. These diets can be particularly helpful for people who have insulin resistance or find carb restriction improves symptoms.

Caution: ketogenic diets require monitoring for nutrient balance, and they're not suitable for everyone (pregnancy, some kidney or liver conditions, history of eating disorders).

3) Anti-inflammatory / low-processed diets (a practical hybrid)

What it looks like: focus on whole foods, eliminate ultra-processed foods and refined sugars, emphasize omega-3 fatty acids, polyphenol-rich plants, and moderate protein.

Why it helps: many lipedema-focused supplement reviews and small interventional studies identify reductions in pain and swelling when diets reduce pro-inflammatory foods and increase antioxidant intake. These approaches are flexible and can be adapted into Mediterranean, plant-forward, or lower-carb patterns.

Key nutrients and supplements — evidence and practical dosing notes

A number of specific nutrients have generated interest and some supportive data. None are magic bullets, but many are reasonable adjuncts when chosen thoughtfully and under clinician guidance.

Omega-3 polyunsaturated fatty acids (EPA/DHA)

Why they help: omega-3s lower inflammatory cytokines and support endothelial and microvascular function — both relevant to the tissue changes seen in lipedema.

Evidence: reviews and supplement analyses consistently point to omega-3 fish oil as one of the most promising adjuncts for symptom reduction and improved inflammatory profiles in lipedema and related adipose disorders.

Practical dosing: many studies use 1–3 g combined EPA+DHA daily. Choose high-quality, third-party tested products and discuss bleeding-risk interactions if you take anticoagulants.

Curcumin (turmeric extracts)

Why it helps: curcumin has well-documented anti-inflammatory and antioxidant effects and improves markers of metabolic health in several meta-analyses.

Evidence: systematic reviews and meta-analyses show curcumin can improve lipid profiles and reduce inflammatory biomarkers; while direct lipedema trials are sparse, curcumin is biologically plausible as part of an anti-inflammatory strategy.

Practical dosing & absorption: curcumin's bioavailability is low unless formulated (phytosome, piperine, liposomal). Typical studied doses range from 500 mg to 2 g daily of a bioavailable formulation. Avoid high doses without medical advice if you take blood thinners or certain medications.

Vitamin D

Why it helps: vitamin D modulates immune responses and low levels are common in many chronic conditions. Adequate vitamin D supports immune regulation and muscle function.

Evidence: while direct lipedema-specific RCTs are limited, screening and correcting deficiency is standard practice because of wide systemic benefits.

Practical dosing: check serum 25-OH vitamin D and supplement to target 25–50 ng/mL under clinician guidance.

Vitamin C, polyphenols, and antioxidants

Why they help: vitamin C supports collagen and capillary health (potentially relevant to easy bruising), while polyphenols (from berries, olive oil, green tea) reduce oxidative stress and inflammation.

Evidence: reviews of supplements for lipedema consistently highlight vitamin C and polyphenol-rich options (olive polyphenols, green tea catechins) as plausible agents with supportive, if limited, human data.

Practical dosing: aim to meet needs through whole foods; supplement vitamin C cautiously if dietary intake is inadequate (usual supplemental ranges 200–500 mg/day unless deficiency or clinician recommendation).

Flavonoids — diosmin/micronized purified flavonoid fraction (MPFF)

Why they help: flavonoids like diosmin and hesperidin improve microvascular tone and lymphovenous function, reducing feelings of heaviness and cramps in venous disease.

Evidence: robust trials in chronic venous disease show benefits for leg pain, cramps, and edema. While direct lipedema evidence is limited, these vascular agents are commonly used as adjuncts where venous symptoms coexist. A randomized, placebo-controlled trial of low-dose diosmin showed symptomatic improvements in venous disease.

Practical dosing: formulations like micronized purified flavonoid fraction (e.g., Daflon®) have standardized dosing; discuss use with a vascular clinician because formulations, dosing, and interactions vary.

Other agents with emerging interest

- **Green tea polyphenols (EGCG):** antioxidant effects; plausible benefits for inflammation.
- **Beta-sitosterol and plant sterols:** discussed in small lipedema supplement reviews for lipid modulation.

- **Magnesium and B vitamins:** helpful for muscle cramps and energy; correct deficiencies as needed.
- **Probiotics / gut health:** theoretical links between microbiome, inflammation, and adipose behavior are being investigated, but robust lipedema data are not yet available.

What the research says about complete dietary programs

A handful of randomized and controlled trials have directly tested dietary interventions in people with lipedema. Recent trials of lower-carbohydrate and ketogenic approaches have reported improvements in pain and quality of life, and reviews note that structured dietary intervention can reduce symptom burden even if limb fat remains. Large, long-term trials are still limited, but the trajectory of evidence supports tailoring diets to reduce inflammation and metabolic stress rather than chasing a single "lipedema diet."

Practical meal planning — making anti-inflammatory eating doable

Below are pragmatic, flexible strategies rather than rigid rules. The goal is sustainability and measurable improvements in how you feel.

Daily priorities

- Vegetables at every meal (leafy greens + colorful vegetables).
- A source of omega-3s twice weekly (fatty fish: salmon, mackerel, sardines) or daily plant sources (chia, flax, walnuts) plus a supplement if needed.
- Replace refined carbs with whole grains or low-carb vegetables depending on your chosen plan.
- Favor extra-virgin olive oil and other minimally processed fats.

- Minimize ultra-processed foods, sugary drinks, and high-salt convenience meals.
- Include a source of lean protein with each meal to stabilize blood sugar and support tissue repair.

A sample day (Mediterranean-informed)

- **Breakfast:** Greek yogurt or unsweetened kefir with berries, ground flaxseed, and a few walnuts.
- **Lunch:** Big salad with mixed greens, chickpeas, grilled salmon (or canned sardines), cherry tomatoes, cucumber, and olive oil + lemon dressing.
- **Snack:** Apple slices with almond butter or carrot sticks and hummus.
- **Dinner:** Roasted vegetables, quinoa or cauliflower rice, and grilled chicken or a hearty lentil stew; finish with a small portion of dark chocolate if desired.
- **Treats:** Use turmeric and ginger in cooking; brew green tea; enjoy dark berries.

For a lower-carb/keto plan, swap grains and starchy vegetables for extra non-starchy veggies and higher-quality fats; prioritize protein and nutrient density, and monitor electrolytes and micronutrients.

Practical shopping list (simple, real-world)

Vegetables: spinach, kale, broccoli, peppers, carrots, zucchini, cruciferous veggies.
Fruits: berries, cherries, citrus (moderate portions if on low-carb).
Proteins: fatty fish, chicken, turkey, legumes (if not carb-restricted), eggs.
Fats: extra-virgin olive oil, avocado, olives, nuts, seeds, fish oil

supplement.
Pantry: quinoa or brown rice (if not low-carb), canned sardines, herbs and spices (turmeric, ginger, black pepper).
Beverages: water, herbal teas, green tea.

Safety, interactions, and special situations

- **Discuss supplements with your clinician.** Omega-3s and curcumin can interact with blood thinners; diosmin and other flavonoids have specific dosing considerations.
- **Pregnancy and breastfeeding:** avoid many supplements or restrictive diets unless supervised by an obstetric clinician and dietitian.
- **Diabetes, kidney disease, or other chronic illnesses:** ketogenic or other restrictive dietary patterns require close monitoring.
- **Allergies and intolerances:** plan substitutions (e.g., plant-based omega-3s if fish allergy).

How to measure progress (meaningful outcomes)

Rather than judging success by limb inches alone, track multiple outcomes:

- **Symptom scores:** pain, heaviness, bruising frequency (use a simple daily log).
- **Function and activity:** number of minutes walked or level of daily tasks you can perform.
- **Quality of life:** sleep quality, mood, energy.

- **Objective metabolic markers:** fasting glucose/HbA1c, lipid panel, vitamin D levels (as indicated).
- Body composition and weight for overall health, not for proving lipedema reversal.

Clinical studies track pain and quality-of-life improvements and show that people can feel markedly better even when limb proportions change little.

Common myths and honest answers

- **Myth: "There is one lipedema diet that cures the disease."** There isn't. Evidence supports inflammation-focused, individualized nutrition as part of overall care.
- **Myth: "Supplements replace the need for medical care."** Supplements are adjuncts; compression, lymphatic care, and medical follow-up remain central.
- **Myth: "If I don't see immediate fat loss, I'm failing."** Fat distribution in lipedema is resistant to diet-only approaches; symptom improvement is a more realistic short-term goal.

Working with professionals — who to involve

- **Registered dietitian (RD)** experienced in inflammatory/metabolic conditions or complex chronic conditions.
- **Primary care clinician** for baseline labs and medication review.
- **Lipedema-aware specialist** (vascular, lymphology, or a lipedema clinic) if available, for coordinated care.

- **Physical therapist** to design exercise that complements diet and compression.

Research frontiers — what to watch for

The nutrition literature for lipedema is growing. Key research areas include:

- Trials comparing Mediterranean vs. low-carb/keto approaches for pain and quality of life.
- Larger, longer RCTs of omega-3s, curcumin, and flavonoids (diosmin) specifically in lipedema populations.
- Mechanistic work linking diet, gut microbiota, and local adipose inflammation in lipedema.

A two-month plan you can try (practical)

Weeks 0–2: Switch to whole foods, remove sugary drinks and ultra-processed snacks, add two omega-3 servings weekly (or supplement), and increase vegetables. Track pain and energy daily.

Weeks 3–6: Choose a pattern (Mediterranean or low-carb) and commit for 4–6 weeks. Add turmeric in cooking daily and consider a curated curcumin supplement if no contraindications. Check vitamin D and correct deficiency.

Weeks 7–8: Review with your RD/clinician: labs, symptom trends, and adjust. Consider adding diosmin or other vascular agents if venous symptoms coexist and under specialist advice.

Questions to bring to your clinician or dietitian

- Is it safe for me to try a low-carb or ketogenic plan given my medical history?
- Should I start omega-3, curcumin, or diosmin? Are there interactions with my medications?
- What baseline labs would you recommend (lipids, glucose, vitamin D, thyroid)?
- Can you refer me to an RD experienced with lipedema or an interdisciplinary clinic?

Closing — food as medicine, not miracle

Nutrition won't erase the structural realities of lipedema, but it is a powerful lever for reducing inflammation, improving energy, and supporting other therapies that together change daily life. The best plan is individualized, realistic, and sustainable: food that you enjoy, that reduces inflammatory load, supports vascular and lymphatic health, and helps you feel stronger and less in pain. Emerging research supports omega-3s, curcumin, and anti-inflammatory dietary patterns as useful tools; careful collaboration with health professionals keeps that approach safe and targeted.

Chapter 7 — Exercise and Physical Therapy

When someone first hears **"exercise"** as part of lipedema care, the reaction is often mixed: hopeful, wary, even angry. Hopeful because movement can relieve pain and improve mood; wary because many people with lipedema have been told "just exercise" as if that alone will fix everything; angry because previous attempts caused more pain or discouragement. This chapter is written for the person who wants a plan that's realistic, safe, and actually helpful — a plan built on how lymphatic physiology, altered adipose tissue, and joint load interact in lipedema, and on the best clinical evidence we have today.

I'll explain the principles behind exercise for lipedema, the types of movement that reliably help (and why), how physical therapists design safe programs, the role of lymphatic drainage and breathing, practical sample sessions and a 12-week plan, common pitfalls, and what the research actually shows. Wherever a claim benefits from a reference, I'll point you to studies and reviews so you — or your clinician — can read deeper. For some influential work on physiotherapy and device-assisted therapies see the randomized trial by Rainer Schneider and for practical therapeutic outlines see the online reference from Physio-Pedia. The manual approach to lymphatic stimulation was pioneered by Emil Vodder, and many clinical summaries live on resources such as the NCBI Bookshelf.

Why exercise matters in lipedema — the physiologic logic

Exercise is not prescribed to "burn off" lipedema fat — that expectation sets people up for disappointment. Instead, exercise helps in several reliable ways:

1. **Activates the muscle pump** — muscle contractions compress veins and lymphatics, helping move blood and lymph centrally and reducing tissue fluid stasis. This is a core reason low-impact movement reduces the heavy, aching feeling many people with lipedema describe. Evidence reviews and clinical guidance identify muscle-activating exercises (walking, swimming, targeted strengthening) as key elements of conservative care.
2. **Improves microvascular and metabolic health** — regular exercise benefits endothelial function, reduces systemic inflammation, and improves metabolic markers that indirectly lower symptom burden. Recent reviews on exercise as a therapeutic tool for lipedema note these effects and suggest exercise is disease-supportive.
3. **Builds functional strength and reduces joint load** — improving core and lower limb strength helps posture and gait, reducing compensatory pain that stems from carrying disproportionate limb mass. Clinical pilot studies and trials of physical therapy protocols report gains in function and reduced pain scores.
4. **Supports lymphatic health when combined with compression and manual therapies** — exercise plus compression or manual lymphatic drainage (MLD) provides

greater short-term improvements in limb volume and symptoms than either alone in several studies.

These mechanisms explain why exercise is a cornerstone of conservative care: it reduces symptoms, improves mobility and quality of life, and prepares patients for other interventions if needed.

What types of exercise help — the practical menu

In lipedema, the best activities share some features: low impact, promote steady muscle-pump activity, avoid excessive eccentric/jarring forces that aggravate joints, and are sustainable. Here's a prioritized list with why and how to do them.

1. Aquatic exercise / hydrotherapy

Why: water's hydrostatic pressure acts like a natural, gentle compression; buoyancy reduces joint load and allows fuller range-of-motion; water resistance builds strength with low impact. **Evidence:** studies of water-based exercise in lymphedema and related conditions report reductions in limb symptoms and improved quality of life; clinicians commonly recommend water-based programs for lipedema because of the dual benefits.

How to start: water walking or aqua aerobics, 30–45 minutes, 2–4x/week. Use shallow or chest-deep water so you can walk briskly and perform gentle kicks, squats, and arm movements.

2. Walking (progressive)

Why: walking activates the calf muscle pump (critical for venous and lymphatic return), is easy to dose, and supports cardiovascular health.
How: start with 10–15 minutes at a comfortable pace, building 5 minutes per week toward 30–45 minutes most days. Use good shoes and compression garments as recommended.

3. Cycling / stationary bike / elliptical

Why: continuous leg-driven movement provides a rhythmic muscle pump with minimal impact on knees and hips.
How: 20–45 minutes, 2–4x/week. Adjust seat and pedal resistance to avoid overloading joints.

4. Strength training (functional, low-to-moderate load)

Why: builds muscle mass, improves posture, and supports joint stability — all crucial when limb mass is disproportionate. Strength training also improves insulin sensitivity and metabolic health.
How: two sessions/week focusing on major patterns (squat/hinge, push/pull, core). Start with bodyweight or light weights, 2–3 sets of 8–15 reps, progress slowly.

5. Yoga / Pilates / mobility and core work

Why: these practices build core stability, improve breath patterns (helpful for lymph flow), reduce stress, and enhance proprioception.
How: focus on gentle sequences and breathing; classes specifically emphasizing therapeutic movement are ideal.

6. Low-frequency vibration and whole-body vibration (WBV) — adjuncts, not standalones

Why: controlled evidence shows low-frequency vibration can augment MLD and improve symptoms in some patients; WBV has anecdotal and some mechanistic support for improving circulation and muscle activation. A randomized pragmatic trial found that low-frequency vibrotherapy improved the effectiveness of manual lymphatic drainage in lipedema.

How to use: under clinician guidance and as an adjunct to exercise and MLD; follow device protocols and start with short sessions (e.g., 10–15 minutes) while monitoring tolerance.

Exercise prescription — practical parameters

A meaningful, safe prescription balances frequency, intensity, time, and type (the FITT principle), and includes progression guidelines.

- **Frequency:** aim for most days of the week for aerobic activity (≥150 min/week moderate intensity spread across 3–5 sessions) and 2 sessions/week of resistance training. For many with lipedema, starting with 3 days/week and gradually increasing is sensible.
- **Intensity:** moderate — you should be able to talk while exercising but not sing. Use perceived exertion (3–5/10) as a practical tool. Avoid repeated high-impact or maximal lifts early on.
- **Time:** start small (10–15 minutes) and increase by 5–10 minutes per session/week until reaching 30–45 minutes.
- **Type:** prioritize low-impact aerobic + functional resistance + mobility + breathing work. Include periodic supervised sessions with a physiotherapist during the first 4–12 weeks.

Progression rule of thumb: increase one variable at a time (time → frequency → intensity) and allow 1–2 weeks at each new level to assess symptom response. If pain or increased swelling persists beyond 48–72 hours, reduce the new load and consult your therapist.

Lymphatic drainage techniques and breathing — what to pair with exercise

Exercise is most effective when paired with lymphatic-supportive practices: diaphragmatic breathing, manual lymphatic drainage (MLD), and simple self-MLD routines.

Diaphragmatic breathing

Why: diaphragmatic (deep belly) breathing creates pressure gradients between thorax and abdomen that promote central lymph flow. It's an easy, low-risk practice to use before and after exercise.
Technique: seated or lying, inhale for 3–4 seconds filling the belly, pause 1–2 seconds, and exhale for 4–6 seconds. Repeat 8–12 breaths as a warm-up.

Manual lymphatic drainage (MLD) and Simple Lymphatic Drainage (SLD)

MLD is a specialized, light massage performed by trained therapists to stimulate lymph flow; SLD is a simplified self-massage patients can learn for daily maintenance. The classic Vodder technique (gentle, rhythmic strokes, proximal-to-distal sequencing) is widely taught and used. Evidence is mixed about MLD alone, but when combined with compression and exercise it often improves symptoms and limb volumes.

Practical steps to learn SLD: a certified therapist teaches sequences to open proximal drainage pathways (neck, groin), then moves lymph from distal limbs toward those pathways using light, skin-stretching strokes. Daily 10–20 minute SLD sessions are common.

Combining MLD with exercise

Many clinics schedule MLD before exercise to open lymphatic pathways and again after exercise to consolidate drainage. Studies show MLD plus pneumatic or vibration devices and exercise produce larger short-term reductions in limb fluid measures than exercise alone.

The role of the physical therapist (PT) and interdisciplinary care

A PT with experience in lymphedema/lipedema is invaluable. Their role may include:

- Detailed baseline assessment (posture, gait, joint ROM, strength, edema distribution).
- Designing and supervising an individualized exercise program that respects pain thresholds and joint issues.
- Teaching SLD and breathing techniques.
- Coordinating compression use (type, timing around exercise).
- Reassessing and progressing the program every 4–6 weeks.

Where available, team care with a vascular specialist, lymphedema therapist, nutritionist, and a surgeon experienced in lipedema produces the best long-term outcomes. Evidence-based guidelines commonly recommend combined approaches (exercise + compression + MLD/CDT) as the core conservative strategy.

Sample session and 12-week starter plan

Below is a practical, clinician-friendly program you can adapt. Check with your clinician before starting.

Sample single session (45 minutes)

1. **Warm-up & breathing (5–8 min):** diaphragmatic breathing + gentle marching on spot.
2. **Aquatic or land aerobic (20 min):** water walk or brisk walking/elliptical at moderate intensity.
3. **Strength circuit (10–12 min):** 2 rounds of 6–8 each: sit-to-stand, band rows, hip bridges, wall push-ups, standing calf raises. Slow, controlled.
4. **Mobility & core (5–8 min):** pelvic tilts, dead bugs, gentle hamstring stretch.
5. **Cool-down & SLD (5–10 min):** gentle walking, diaphragmatic breathing, and a short self-MLD routine.

12-week progression (starter)

- **Weeks 1–4:** 3 sessions/week (2 structured + 1 light active day). Focus: build tolerance, learn breathing/SLD.
- **Weeks 5–8:** 3–4 sessions/week. Increase aerobic duration to 30 min; add light resistance and 1 focused mobility class (yoga/Pilates). Consider 1 supervised PT session/week for technique.
- **Weeks 9–12:** 4–5 sessions/week: 2 aerobic (30–45 min), 2 strength (20–30 min), 1 mobility/recovery. Introduce interval walking (light) if tolerated and continue SLD daily. Assess outcomes at week 12 (pain, function, QoL).

Adapt intensity and volume to symptoms — the aim is consistent, progressive gains without prolonged flare.

Red flags, contraindications, and when to slow down

Exercise is generally safe, but watch for:

- **New or worsening pitting edema, increasing pain, or skin changes** — consult clinician; may indicate lymphatic overload or infection.
- **Infection (cellulitis)** — do not exercise the affected limb until cleared by a provider.
- **Severe joint instability or acute injury** — modify or avoid weightbearing; use water therapy or cycling.
- **Cardiovascular limitations or pregnancy** — get medical clearance and adapt intensity.

If a new exercise leads to persistent worsening for >72 hours, reduce load and consult your PT.

Evidence summary — what the research tells us

- **Exercise reduces symptoms and improves function:** systematic reviews and trials show exercise programs improve pain, quality of life, limb circumference, and functional performance in women with lipedema; effects are more consistent when compression is used concurrently.
- **Physical therapy shows promise in early disease:** pilot and proof-of-principle PT studies in early lipedema report improved outcomes with targeted programs.

- **Adjunct devices aid outcomes:** low-frequency vibration has RCT evidence of augmenting MLD effectiveness; pneumatic devices and WBV have promising mechanistic and small clinical data but need larger trials.
- **Hydrotherapy is beneficial for symptom relief and mobility:** water programs are supported by lymphedema literature and practical clinic use for lipedema.
- In short: exercise is evidence-based for symptom relief and function, but the most robust improvements occur within combined, individualized programs.

Practical tips for adherence and long-term success

1. **Start small and celebrate consistency** — frequent short sessions beat epic one-offs.
2. **Choose enjoyable activities** — social walking groups, aquatic classes, or gentle yoga increase adherence.
3. **Use compression strategically** — many people feel better exercising with compression garments that fit well.
4. **Track outcomes beyond inches** — mood, sleep, pain, and minutes of activity matter.
5. **Build a team** — a PT, lymph therapist, and supportive clinician help troubleshoot and maintain progress.

Future directions and research needs

Researchers are actively testing comparative diet + exercise programs, device-assisted adjuncts (WBV, pneumatic), and optimal dosing of MLD combined with exercise. Larger randomized trials and standardized outcome sets are necessary to refine best-practice exercise prescriptions — but the current evidence already supports exercise as a central, practical therapy for symptom control and functional improvement.

Movement as medicine, adapted and humane

Exercise for lipedema should never feel like punishment or a demand to "fix" your body. It's a tool to reduce pain, improve mobility, and increase your agency. A good program is individualized, starts from where you are, progresses slowly, and respects the reality of tender tissue and joint strain. Work with a therapist who understands lipedema when you can, pair movement with breathing, compression, and self-MLD, and prioritize consistency over intensity. Over time, small, steady gains in function and comfort add up — and that's what changes daily life.

Chapter 8 — Liposuction for Lipedema

Lipedema is stubborn in ways that go beyond body shape: it can be painful, limiting, and psychologically heavy. For many people with advanced or refractory symptoms, liposuction is the first time they experience a true, measurable improvement in pain, mobility, and daily comfort. But—from the patient's point of view—liposuction for lipedema is not the same as cosmetic liposuction. It's a therapeutic, carefully staged intervention with its own rules, risks, and long-term care needs. This chapter explains, in plain language and with clinical perspective, what lipedema liposuction is, how it's done, when it helps, what the evidence and limitations are, how to choose a surgeon and prepare for surgery, common complications and how they're managed, and what life looks like after the procedure.

What liposuction for lipedema aims to do (and what it does not)

Therapeutic liposuction for lipedema is designed to:

- Remove pathological subcutaneous fat that causes pain, heaviness, and functional impairment.
- Improve limb shape and proportionality to reduce mechanical strain and chafing.

- Reduce symptom burden (pain, tenderness, spontaneous bruising) and often improve mobility and quality of life.

Important caveats to hold from the start: liposuction is **not** a cure. Lipedema is a chronic condition that requires lifelong conservative care (compression, exercise, skin care, lymphatic support) even after surgery. Liposuction reduces the volume and the disease-related symptoms for many patients, but ongoing self-care and follow-up are essential.

Clinical outcomes across multiple series show meaningful symptom and quality-of-life improvements after liposuction, often sustained over months to years in reported cohorts. These findings are supported by patient-reported outcome studies and systematic clinical reviews.

How lipedema liposuction differs from cosmetic liposuction

The approach used for lipedema emphasizes tissue preservation, lymphatic protection, and staged volumes rather than aggressive, single-session body contouring. Key differences:

- **Lymph-sparing technique:** Surgeons use smaller cannulas, gentler aspiration, and techniques that minimize injury to lymphatic collectors (see section below on lymphatic preservation).
- **Staging:** Large treatment areas are often addressed over multiple operative sessions to reduce fluid shifts, blood loss, and swelling.
- **Objective goals:** The primary outcomes are symptom reduction, improved function, and reduced reliance on conservative measures — not merely aesthetic contour.

- **Perioperative plan:** Careful preop assessment, supplies of compression garments, and coordinated postoperative lymphatic and physiotherapy follow-up are routine.

Because of these differences, patient selection and surgeon experience matter a great deal.

Major surgical techniques used today

Several liposuction methods are commonly applied in lipedema management. The methods aim to dislodge and remove diseased fat while minimizing trauma to the lymphatic system.

Tumescent liposuction (fluid injection + suction)

Tumescent liposuction infiltrates a large volume of dilute local anesthetic and epinephrine into the tissues before suctioning. It reduces bleeding and provides local anesthesia, allowing precise suctioning of the subcutaneous fat. This method, when performed carefully with small cannulas and lymph-sparing technique, is widely used for lipedema and favored for its safety profile and tissue preservation.

Water-assisted liposuction (WAL)

Water-assisted liposuction uses a pressurized saline stream to gently dislodge fat cells before aspiration. Multiple clinical series report WAL to be efficient at removing lipedema fat while preserving connective tissue and lymphatic structures when used by experienced teams. Early and mid-term outcome studies report sustained reduction of disease-related complaints with WAL when performed in specialized centers.

Super-wet and other variations

"Super-wet" uses smaller fluid volumes than classic tumescent techniques and may shorten operative time. The key across all approaches is skilled, gentle technique and the use of appropriate cannula sizes and trajectories to avoid lymphatic injury.

Lymphatic preservation — what it means and how it's achieved

A central tenet of modern lipedema surgery is lymphatic preservation. Damaging lymphatic collectors during aggressive fat removal can lead to or worsen lymphedema, which substantially complicates recovery and long-term function. Surgeons who specialize in lipedema focus on:

- **Gentle traction and small cannulas** to reduce trauma.
- **Shallow suction planes** that preferentially remove superficial diseased fat rather than deep tissue close to lymphatic collectors.
- **Intraoperative lymphatic mapping** using indocyanine green (ICG) fluorescence in selected centers to identify and avoid important lymphatic channels during the procedure. Early series of ICG-guided approaches demonstrate that real-time visualization can help spare lymphatics while achieving debulking goals.

If you are considering surgery, ask the surgeon whether they routinely perform lymphatic-sparing techniques and whether they use intraoperative mapping like ICG.

Who is a good candidate?

Ideal surgical candidates usually have:

- Clinically diagnosed lipedema with documented symptoms (pain, tenderness, functional limitation) that have not adequately responded to conservative measures (compression, MLD, physiotherapy).
- Realistic expectations: improvement in pain and mobility, reduction in limb size, but an understanding that lifelong conservative care remains needed.
- Medical fitness for anesthesia and staged surgical treatment, as determined after preoperative evaluation.

Patients with severe lymphatic failure (advanced lipolymphedema), uncontrolled medical comorbidities, or active infection need careful multidisciplinary evaluation. Many centers prefer to treat earlier disease stages because outcomes and lymphatic preservation are often better when the tissue is less fibrotic.

What the evidence says — benefits and limitations

The growing body of literature, including systematic reviews and patient-reported outcome studies, indicates that liposuction for lipedema can:

- Reduce pain and spontaneous tenderness.
- Improve mobility and ease of movement.
- Improve quality of life in many patients, with patient-reported benefits documented months to years after surgery.

Limitations and unknowns remain:

- Long-term, randomized controlled trials comparing surgical and non-surgical care are limited; much of the evidence is observational or from before-after studies. Systematic scoping reviews emphasize beneficial effects but call for more standardized long-term outcome data.

This is why choosing an experienced center that tracks outcomes and participates in registries or studies is advantageous — it both improves your care and contributes to the evidence base.

Risks and complications — what to know (and how common they are)

Like any surgery, liposuction carries risks. Some are shared with cosmetic liposuction; others are specific to lipedema patients due to lymphatic vulnerability or treatment of large volumes.

Key potential complications include:

- **Fluid imbalance and bleeding:** careful fluid management is essential perioperatively.
- **Fat embolism and thromboembolic events (DVT/PE):** large-volume liposuction carries a non-zero risk of fat embolism and venous thromboembolism; vigilant intraoperative technique and postoperative prophylaxis are important. Systematic safety reviews emphasize these rare but serious risks and the need for appropriate patient selection and monitoring.
- **Infection and wound problems:** rates vary; wound infection and erysipelas have been reported and require prompt treatment.
- **Asymmetry or contour irregularities:** staged treatments and meticulous technique reduce these risks.

- **Lymphatic injury and new or worsened lymphedema:** the most feared complication in this population — this is why lymph-sparing approaches and surgeon experience matter greatly.

Complication rates reported in the literature vary by center, technique, and patient selection; experienced centers report acceptable complication profiles when strict lymph-preserving techniques and staged protocols are used.

Preparing for surgery — checklist and practical advice

Good outcomes begin before the day of surgery. Practical preoperative steps include:

1. **Comprehensive medical evaluation** — labs, anesthetic assessment, optimization of comorbid conditions (blood pressure, glucose control, smoking cessation).
2. **Compression and physiotherapy planning** — secure post-op compression garments in advance and coordinate with your lymphatic therapist or physical therapist for postoperative drainage and exercise. Postoperative compression is a crucial component of recovery and skin retraction.
3. **Medication review** — stop or adjust medications that increase bleeding risk (anticoagulants, some supplements) only with medical guidance.
4. **Logistics:** arrange for someone to drive you home and help for the first 48–72 hours; set up a comfortable recovery area with easy access to fluids, dressing supplies, and prescribed medications.

5. **Realistic planning:** most centers plan multiple staged procedures for large-area disease; discuss the number and timing of stages and expected time off work.

Ask your surgeon for written protocols about preop fasting, which medications to avoid, and the expected timeline for each stage.

The operation and immediate recovery

Typical perioperative themes:

- **Anesthesia:** procedures may be performed under local tumescent anesthesia with sedation, regional blocks, or general anesthesia depending on volume and patient comfort.
- **Staging & volumes:** surgeons often limit suction volumes per session to safer thresholds and perform sequential procedures (legs in one stage, arms in another, etc.).
- **Compression & drains:** many surgeons use immediate compression garments and sometimes drains (practice varies). Close follow-up is usual in the first two weeks to monitor swelling, wound healing, and any signs of complications.
- **Pain & swelling:** expect bruising and swelling that peaks in the first week and gradually reduces over several weeks to months. Pain is usually manageable with prescribed analgesics and supportive care.

Postoperative care — the first weeks and months

Post-op care is central to success and includes:

- **Compression:** wear prescribed compression continuously (except for gentle washing) for the initial weeks; transition schedules vary but most protocols move toward daytime wear for months afterward. Compression supports skin retraction and reduces bruising and edema.

- **Manual lymphatic drainage (MLD) and self-care:** MLD (provided by a certified therapist) and taught self-MLD techniques are commonly used to move fluid and speed recovery. The history and rationale of MLD go back to the Vodder method (Emil Vodder and colleagues), and many lipedema teams integrate MLD into postoperative plans.
- **Gradual return to activity:** walking is encouraged early; driving, heavy lifting, and strenuous exercise are delayed according to the surgeon's timeline (often several weeks to months for full intensity training).
- **Skin and wound care:** follow instructions for dressing changes and infection signs; early treatment of any erysipelas or cellulitis is critical.
- **Follow-up and scar management:** routine clinic visits at 1–2 weeks, 6 weeks, and periodic assessments thereafter help catch and manage complications early.

Be sure you have clear written instructions and contact numbers for the surgical team in case concerns arise.

Long-term outcomes and realistic expectations

Many people experience sustained improvements in pain, bruising frequency, ease of movement, and overall quality of life after liposuction for lipedema — often after several stages and with ongoing conservative care. However:

- **Recurrence and new fat accumulation:** while liposuction removes pathological fat in treated areas, fat can still accumulate in untreated areas and weight changes may alter distribution.
- **Lifelong management:** continued compression during high-risk times, adherence to exercise, and attention to skin health remain part of long-term care.
- **Surgical results and satisfaction:** high patient satisfaction is reported in many series when expectations are realistic and care is multidisciplinary.

Choosing a surgeon and center that tracks functional and patient-reported outcomes transparently will give you the best sense of likely results for your situation.

Choosing a surgeon and center — important questions to ask

When evaluating a surgeon or clinic, consider asking:

- How many lipedema-specific liposuction procedures do you perform per year?
- Do you use lymph-sparing techniques, and can you describe your approach?
- Do you use intraoperative lymphatic mapping such as ICG? If so, how often and in which patients?
- Can you share patient outcome data or references from recent patients (anonymized)?
- What is your staged treatment protocol for large areas?
- Who coordinates postoperative MLD, compression fitting, and rehabilitation?
- What is your complication rate and how do you manage complications like infection or DVT?

A transparent surgeon will provide clear answers, written protocols, and references or outcome summaries.

Common patient questions — frank answers

Will I be "fixed" after liposuction?
No. Many people gain substantial symptom relief, but lipedema is a chronic condition requiring ongoing management.

Is it painful?
Surgical discomfort is expected, but modern techniques, anesthesia options, and multimodal pain control typically make the immediate postoperative period manageable.

How many sessions will I need?
It depends on the extent of disease. Many patients require staged procedures (two to four sessions is not uncommon for widespread disease), spaced months apart.

Will insurance cover it?
Coverage varies widely by country, insurer, and documentation of medical necessity. Increasingly, insurers recognize therapeutic liposuction for lipedema when conservative measures have failed, but prior authorization and detailed documentation are often needed.

Red flags and when to seek urgent care

After surgery, contact your surgeon or seek urgent care for:

- Sudden shortness of breath, chest pain, or signs of pulmonary embolism.

- Rapidly increasing pain, high fever, or spreading redness (possible deep infection).
- New neurological symptoms or sudden severe limb swelling that's asymmetric.

Early detection of complications is essential to prevent serious outcomes.

Research frontiers — what's next for lipedema surgery

Active areas of research and innovation include:

- **ICG-guided lymphatic identification** to further reduce lymphatic injury risk.
- **Comparative outcomes of WAL vs tumescent vs other techniques**, with attention to long-term function and recurrence.
- **Standardized outcome measures** and registries to permit robust comparisons across centers and to better document long-term benefits and risks.

As research matures, surgical protocols will continue to evolve toward safer, more durable outcomes.

Final thoughts — a balanced, informed choice

For many people with symptomatic lipedema, liposuction is life-changing: pain diminishes, mobility improves, and everyday life becomes easier. But the decision to move forward should be informed, staged, and supported by a multidisciplinary team: an experienced lymphatic or lipedema surgeon, a certified lymphatic therapist, knowledgeable physiotherapists, and primary care support. Ask about lymph-sparing techniques, staged approaches, postoperative compression and MLD plans, complication rates, and the team's outcome data. When chosen and performed thoughtfully, lipedema-focused liposuction is a powerful therapeutic option — not a miracle cure, but a durable step toward better quality of life.

Chapter 9 — Post-Surgical Care

Undergoing liposuction for lipedema is often a turning point: pain eases, mobility improves, and daily life becomes easier. But the operation is just one step. Recovery — the hours, days, weeks, and months afterward — is where the long-term benefits are secured (or lost). This chapter walks you through realistic expectations, step-by-step care, evidence-informed practices, and the common problems people face after lipedema surgery. My goal is to translate clinical practice into an accessible playbook you can use at home, in the clinic, or to guide questions for your surgical team.

A realistic overview: what surgery does and why aftercare matters

Therapeutic liposuction removes pathological subcutaneous fat and can dramatically reduce pain and improve function. But it also creates trauma to soft tissue: the body responds with inflammation, bruising, and fluid shifts. How you manage those responses — compression, movement, wound care, lymphatic support, and monitoring for complications — largely determines how quickly you recover and how good the long-term outcomes are. Major centers and clinical reviews emphasize that post-op protocols (compression, early mobilization, lymphatic therapy, DVT prophylaxis when indicated) are essential to safe, effective recovery.

The first 24–72 hours: immediate recovery basics

What to expect

- **Sleep and rest are normal:** anesthesia and opioids make people very sleepy for the first day or two.
- **Drainage and dressings:** small incisions may leak tumescent fluid and blood for the first 24–72 hours; absorbent dressings help manage this.
- **Pain & bruising:** pain is expected but usually controllable with prescribed medications; bruising can be extensive but gradually improves over weeks.
- **Walking:** short, frequent walks the evening of surgery or the next day are encouraged to stimulate circulation and reduce DVT risk — but avoid long standing, heavy lifting, or intense activity. Clinical teams commonly ask patients to start gentle ambulation as soon as safe.

Practical checklist for day-one

- Have your compression garments ready and put them on as your surgeon advises (many centers transition from short-term wraps into fitted garments within 24–48 hours).
- Keep dressings clean and dry; follow instructions about showering.
- Drink water, eat light protein-rich meals, and avoid alcohol while taking pain meds.
- Arrange help for the first 48–72 hours (driving, childcare, grocery runs).

Compression: timing, types, and how long to wear it

Why it matters

Compression reduces edema, supports tissue re-approximation, and helps skin retract. For lipedema patients, compression is both a short-term support after surgery and a long-term maintenance strategy. Evidence summaries and specialty guidance recommend wearing properly fitted post-op garments for extended durations tailored to stage and volume removed. Many centers advise continuous compression for the first 2–3 months, with ongoing daytime compression for longer depending on clinical response.

Practical details

- **Immediate phase (0–2 weeks):** surgeons commonly use short-stretch bandaging or temporary compression wraps in the first 24–48 hours, then move to medical-grade garments as wounds permit.
- **Early healing (2–12 weeks):** continuous daytime wear of graduated compression is usually advised; night-time use depends on surgeon preference and garment type.
- **Longer term (after 3 months):** many patients continue daytime compression during periods of prolonged standing, exercise, or travel and may maintain nighttime compression if recommended by their team. The exact duration varies by stage, volumes removed, and individual response.

Fit and function

- Use professionally fitted garments — ill-fitting compression contributes to pressure points, discomfort, and poor results. Ask about flat-knit vs round-knit options if you have uneven shapes or large volumes. Replace garments when elasticity declines (typically every 6–12 months of regular use).

Manual lymphatic drainage (MLD) and self-care lymphatic techniques

What MLD does
MLD is a gentle, rhythmic technique that stimulates lymph flow and reduces fluid accumulation. It's widely used after liposuction to speed reduction of edema and minimize fibrosis (scar tissue formation). Many surgeons and clinics incorporate MLD into post-op care, but timing varies with wound healing and surgeon preference.

When to start

- Some centers start very early (48–72 hours) for carefully selected patients, while others prefer waiting 1–2 weeks until the initial wound drainage and acute inflammation subside. The safest timing and frequency should be individualized and determined by your surgical and lymphatic therapy teams.

Self-MLD and breathing

- Therapists typically teach a short daily self-MLD routine (10–20 minutes) that opens proximal drainage pathways (neck, groin) first and then moves fluid from distal to proximal. Diaphragmatic breathing is a simple adjunct that promotes central lymph flow and is easy to do before and after sessions.

Mobilization, activity progression, and return to work

The balance to aim for is early movement to prevent complications without overstressing healing tissues.

Early days (0–14 days)

- **Walking:** short, frequent walks multiple times daily to stimulate circulation and avoid clots.
- **No heavy lifting:** avoid lifting >10 pounds (≈4–5 kg) for 2–4 weeks or longer as your surgeon advises.
- **Elevate legs** when resting to reduce dependent swelling. Avoid prolonged standing.

Weeks 2–6

- **Increase low-impact activity:** longer walks, light stationary bike, and gentle range of motion under compression.
- **Begin guided physiotherapy** (if recommended) to restore mobility, gait, and core strength.

After 6–12 weeks

- **Gradual return to higher intensity exercise** (strength, interval work) is possible if swelling, wound healing, and pain are controlled. Always coordinate with your surgical and PT teams.

Return to work

- Desk jobs: many patients return within 1–2 weeks if pain is controlled and mobility is adequate.
- Physically demanding jobs: expect 4–8 weeks or more, depending on job demands and staged treatment.

Pain control: multimodal strategies

Pain after liposuction is expected but usually controllable.

Medication strategies

- **Short courses of opioids** may be prescribed initially for breakthrough pain; rely on them sparingly and taper as able.
- **Scheduled non-opioid analgesics** (acetaminophen ± NSAID if approved by your surgeon) and adjuvants (gabapentin for neuropathic-type pain in some protocols) form the backbone of multimodal analgesia. Surgeons commonly avoid NSAIDs in the immediate perioperative window in some cases due to bleeding concerns — follow your surgeon's guidance.
- **Topical agents** and cold compresses (when advised) can soothe superficial discomfort — be sure to avoid direct ice on high-compression areas or incisions unless instructed.

Non-drug approaches

- Elevation, compression, gentle walking, and MLD reduce pain by lowering edema and tissue tension. Mindful breathing, relaxation, and graded activity help reduce pain perception and improve sleep.

Wound care, infection prevention, and cellulitis risk

Incision care

- Keep incisions clean and dry per your surgeon's instructions. Many teams allow showering after 24–48 hours with specific dressing instructions; avoid soaking or baths until wounds are fully healed.

Signs to watch for

- Increasing redness, spreading warmth, worsening pain, fever, or purulent drainage suggest infection and require prompt medical review. Lipedema patients can be at higher risk for cellulitis; early treatment prevents complications. Clinical teams emphasize quick treatment of erysipelas/cellulitis to prevent deeper tissue involvement.

Antibiotics

- Some surgeons provide a short perioperative antibiotic course; others reserve antibiotics for clear signs of infection. Follow your surgeon's instructions and call early if you suspect infection.

Skin hygiene and long-term vigilance

- Gentle moisturizing of healed skin, monitoring for fissures or intertrigo in skin folds, and rapid treatment of minor breaks reduce infection risk. If you have recurrent cellulitis historically, discuss prophylactic strategies with your team.

Venous thromboembolism (VTE) prevention

Why it's important

- Liposuction — particularly large-volume or staged operations — carries VTE risk. Prevention is a major safety focus and includes risk stratification (Caprini score or equivalent) and perioperative measures. Evidence reviews in plastic surgery recommend mechanical and, for many patients, pharmacologic prophylaxis tailored to risk.

Common measures

- **Early ambulation** is essential.
- **Mechanical prophylaxis:** sequential compression devices in hospital and graduated compression at home.
- **Chemical prophylaxis:** low-molecular-weight heparin (e.g., enoxaparin) is commonly used in higher-risk patients, with start times and duration individualized to bleeding risk and surgeon preference. Clinical guidance suggests chemoprophylaxis timing (often starting 6–12 hours post-op in many protocols) and potentially extending prophylaxis for weeks in high-risk cases.

Discuss your personal VTE risk with your surgeon before the operation, and plan for the agreed prophylaxis regimen.

Swelling timeline, fibrosis, and what to expect cosmetically

Typical course

- **Weeks 0–2:** Peak swelling and bruising.
- **Weeks 3–12:** Gradual reduction of edema; contours become clearer though firmness and numbness may persist.
- **Months 3–12:** Continued remodeling, skin retraction, and softening of fibrotic areas; scars mature and fade.

Fibrosis and scar tissue

- Untreated fibrosis can limit contour outcomes and comfort. Early MLD, compression, and physiotherapy reduce the risk of excessive fibrosis. If stubborn fibrosis develops, some centers use targeted massage, physiotherapy techniques, or in rare cases secondary interventions.

Patience and realistic expectations

- Final results can take many months. Expect incremental improvement and plan staged procedures and rehabilitation accordingly.

Emotional and psychological recovery

Surgery touches identity and body image. Many patients feel elated by reduced pain and mobility; others experience unexpected emotional waves during recovery (vulnerability, body image shifts, temporary dependence). Prepare for this:

- Arrange social support and realistic help at home.
- Consider counseling or peer support groups for lipedema patients who have undergone surgery — hearing others' journeys normalizes the process.
- Discuss expectations candidly with your surgical team beforehand; clear, realistic goals reduce postoperative disappointment.

Preparing your home and caregivers

Make the first week comfortable:

- Soft pillows and leg elevation supplies.
- Easy-reach healthy snacks and protein-rich foods.
- A place with minimal stair use if mobility will be limited.
- A phone list with your surgeon, clinic nurse, and emergency contacts.
- Assistive tools (grabber, slip-on shoes, dressing aids) and a plan for help with chores and children/pets.

When to call your surgeon — red flags

Seek urgent care or call your surgical team for:

- Shortness of breath, chest pain, or rapid heartbeat (possible pulmonary embolism).
- New or worsening unilateral leg swelling, severe pain, or calf tenderness (possible DVT).
- Rapidly spreading redness, high fever, severe pain, or purulent drainage (possible serious infection).
- Uncontrolled bleeding or sudden, severe bruising beyond expected levels.

Long-term maintenance after recovery

Surgery reduces pathological fat in treated areas, but it's part of a lifelong management plan:

- **Compression:** continue as advised, especially during prolonged standing, flights, and exercise.
- **Exercise and PT:** maintain a tailored exercise plan to support circulation and strength.
- **Skin care and infection prevention:** daily attention prevents complications.
- **Follow-up:** periodic clinic visits to check scars, lymphatic function, and overall satisfaction — and to plan any additional staged procedures if needed.

Evidence and outcomes — what the literature says briefly

Clinical series and systematic reviews report meaningful reductions in pain, improved mobility, and better quality of life after lipedema-focused liposuction performed with lymph-sparing techniques. Yet randomized long-term trials remain limited; therefore experienced centers stress careful selection, staged operations, and multidisciplinary aftercare to optimize outcomes and minimize complications.

Practical patient checklist — the essentials

Before surgery

- Confirm surgeon experience with lipedema and lymph-sparing technique.
- Arrange post-op compression and lymphatic therapy appointments.
- Plan transport and home support for 48–72 hours.

First 48–72 hours

- Wear compression as instructed; begin short walks; manage dressings per instructions; hydrate and eat protein.

Weeks 1–6

- Start MLD or SLD when cleared; continue compression; begin guided PT and gradually increase activity.

Weeks 6–12+

- Transition to tailored exercise; discuss longer-term compression schedules; monitor scars, function, and any infection signs.

Long term

- Maintain exercise, compression during risk periods, skin care, and periodical follow-up.

Final thoughts — teamwork and realistic care

The surgical event is a powerful tool for reducing lipedema symptoms, but the "after" is where most of the work — and the benefit — lies. A thoughtful plan that combines compression, early mobilization, careful wound care, lymphatic support, VTE prevention, and staged rehabilitation will give you the best chance of lasting benefit. Ask for clear, written postoperative instructions, confirm the roles of your surgical, lymphatic, and physiotherapy team, and keep a low threshold for contacting your clinic about any worrying sign. Recovery is rarely a straight line — setbacks can happen, but with good team support and steady self-care, most people reach meaningful, durable improvements in comfort and function.

Part III: Living with Lipedema

Chapter 10 — Psychological Impact and Support

Lipedema reaches deeper than the skin. It shows up in everyday tasks, in how you see yourself in the mirror, and in the quiet moments when your body refuses to do what you want it to. That physical reality invites a lot of emotional work — grief for the body you expected, frustration at misdiagnosis, exhaustion from constant management, and sometimes panic or despair over the social costs. This chapter is written for the person who needs both validation and practical tools: I'll explain the common emotional reactions, what the research tells us about mental-health burden, how to find the right kinds of psychological help, practical coping strategies you can use today, and how families and clinicians can become effective allies.

The emotional truth of living with lipedema

Lipedema is experienced, for many people, as a chronic, often invisible burden. The physical symptoms — pain, heaviness, gait changes, repeated skin infections — are plainly distressing. But there are other layers that often hurt just as much.

- **Identity and body image.** For many, lipedema changes the body in ways that clash with personal or social ideals of attractiveness and health. That can result in body-checking, avoidance of social situations, and a fractured relationship with movement and food. Studies document significant body-image disturbance in lipedema populations.

- **Shame and blame.** Because lipedema is commonly mislabelled as simple obesity, many patients internalize messages that their condition is due to laziness or lack of willpower. That internalized stigma fuels depression, anxiety, and avoidance of care. Recent surveys show high rates of perceived weight stigma and internalized weight bias in people living with lipedema, which strongly correlates with depressive symptoms.
- **Practical losses and grief.** Loss of mobility, a shrinking wardrobe, difficulties in intimacy, and limitations at work are real, cumulative losses. Grief about these losses is normal and deserves space and validation. Qualitative work on lived experience across stages of lipedema emphasizes the constant negotiation between acceptance and hope for improvement.
- **Depression and anxiety.** Numerous clinical reviews document elevated rates of anxiety and depressive symptoms among people with lipedema; one authoritative standards-of-care review notes that 42% of people with lipedema showed anxiety or depression on standardized measures and that a large majority report impacts on mental health and self-esteem.

These emotional experiences are not "secondary" or immaterial: they influence help-seeking, adherence to therapies (compression, exercise, nutrition), willingness to consider surgery, and the ability to sustain daily life. Treating lipedema effectively means treating the whole person — body and mind.

Common psychological reactions — what's typical and what's a red flag

Most people with lipedema move through several psychological phases, though the sequence and intensity vary:

1. **Confusion and relief (at diagnosis).** Finally getting a name for symptoms can bring enormous relief — but also the dawning sense that this will be a long road.
2. **Anger and protest.** Anger at earlier misdiagnoses, at clinicians who blamed weight, or at social shaming is common. This anger is a healthy reaction to injustice and can be a mobilizing force for advocacy.
3. **Bargaining and attempts to fix.** Many patients attempt course after course of diet and exercise (sometimes extreme) trying to "fix" what is not simply weight-based fat. That can lead to cycles of hope and disappointment.
4. **Grief and acceptance work.** Over time, many people do grief work around limitations and then pivot toward strategic self-care. For others, chronic depression or anxiety becomes entrenched and needs targeted treatment.
5. **Resilience and activism.** Many people find renewed purpose through peer leadership, advocacy, and helping others navigate care.

Red flags that warrant urgent or specialized attention: suicidal thoughts or plans, severe functional decline from depression (unable to work or care for self), panic attacks that limit leaving home, severe disordered eating, and substance misuse. If any of these occur, seek immediate professional help.

Evidence behind the emotional burden — what studies show

We don't have to rely on anecdotes. Multiple empirical studies and reviews document elevated psychological burden in lipedema:

- Large clinical overviews report higher-than-expected rates of depression and anxiety and widespread reports that lipedema negatively affects mental health and coping.
- Qualitative and survey studies describe the lived experience across disease stages — showing how stigma, delayed diagnosis, and physical limitation combine to reduce health-related quality of life.
- Research on internalized weight bias and stigma in lipedema populations links that stigma to worse depressive symptom scores and lower social participation.

These studies make a practical point: the emotional toll is measurable and common, so routine mental-health screening should be part of lipedema care.

Evidence-based psychological treatments that help

A number of therapeutic approaches show benefit for people with chronic physical conditions and pain; many of these generalize to lipedema.

Cognitive Behavioral Therapy (CBT)

CBT helps people change unhelpful thinking patterns and develop practical coping skills (behavioral activation, pacing, problem-solving). In chronic pain populations, CBT reduces pain-related distress and improves daily functioning; systematic reviews of CBT-based interventions for comorbid psychological distress and pain indicate meaningful benefits. For lipedema patients, CBT can target shame, body-image distortions, and maladaptive health behaviors.

Practical CBT benefits include:

- Reducing catastrophic thinking about pain and disability
- Rebuilding a manageable activity plan (pacing vs. boom-and-bust activity cycles)
- Treating low mood and anxiety with structured behavioral experiments and activity scheduling

Acceptance and Commitment Therapy (ACT)

ACT emphasizes values, psychological flexibility, and living a meaningful life even with ongoing pain or limitations. For people tired of "fixing" and ready to reclaim activities they value, ACT offers a compassionate framework.

Body-image therapies and mirror work

Because body-image disturbance is common, targeted interventions that combine CBT techniques with exposure, self-compassion training, and somatic reconnection exercises can reduce avoidance and improve body acceptance. Evidence in related conditions (e.g., persistent body dissatisfaction) supports these approaches.

Interventions for sleep and insomnia (CBT-I)

Sleep disruption is common in chronic pain and chronic illness. CBT for insomnia (CBT-I) is an evidence-based approach that treats the behaviors and thoughts that maintain poor sleep and can markedly improve sleep without medication. Improved sleep usually helps mood, pain thresholds, and daytime functioning. (CBT-I is recommended first-line for chronic insomnia.)

Group therapy and psychoeducation

Group formats — whether CBT groups, ACT groups, or psychoeducation groups — provide symptom-management training plus the added benefit of peer normalization. For many people with lipedema, group sessions are the first place they hear other patients describe the same misdiagnoses and frustrations; that normalization alone is therapeutic.

Practical psychological tools you can use now

You don't have to wait for therapy to start helpful habits. These are practical, low-risk strategies that many patients find useful.

1. **Daily micro-wins (behavioral activation).** Set one small, achievable activity each day that aligns with your values (e.g., 10 minutes of walking, calling a friend, making one nourishing meal). Win early and build momentum.
2. **Pacing, not pushing.** Track activity and symptoms for a week. Notice patterns of boom-and-bust (crash after a big push). Practice limiting effort to a sustainable baseline and gradually increasing by 10% once stable for a week.
3. **Cognitive reframing for shame.** Notice self-blaming thoughts like "If I were stronger, I wouldn't have this." Ask: "Is that thought fully true? What evidence contradicts it?" Replace with compassionate facts: "This is a medical condition; I am doing the best I can."

4. **Self-MLD and breathing as calming rituals.** Diaphragmatic breathing, followed by a 5–10 minute self-MLD routine (learned from a certified therapist), can reduce bodily tension and cue restful states.
5. **Sleep hygiene and CBT-I basics.** Keep a consistent sleep–wake schedule, avoid screens 60 minutes before bed, use the bed only for sleep/sex, and restrict time in bed to actual sleep time when insomnia is a problem. If sleep does not improve, seek CBT-I.
6. **Compassion practices.** Short guided compassion or mindfulness exercises (5–10 minutes daily) reduce stress and improve emotional resilience.

These tools are low-cost, low-risk, and can be used alongside clinical therapy and medical care.

Peer support: why it matters and how to find it

Feeling alone with a condition that's often misdiagnosed fuels despair. Peer support is one of the highest-value, lowest-cost interventions available.

- **Why it helps:** peer groups reduce isolation, provide practical tips (best compression brands, how to talk to employers), and model successful coping strategies. Many patients report that meeting others with lipedema was the first time they felt believed. (See clinic and advocacy group resources for local groups.)
- **Where to look:** local lymphedema/lipedema clinics often run support groups; national advocacy organizations host moderated online groups and directories. If you prefer

anonymity, moderated online forums and closed social-media groups can be safe starting points.

- **How to get maximum benefit:** choose groups that emphasize evidence-informed information, avoid spaces that promote extreme "cures" or unsupervised medical advice, and consider a short trial of a few groups to find the right fit.

Peer support is not a substitute for professional therapy in the case of severe depression or suicidal ideation, but it is a powerful complement for everyday coping.

When to choose psychotherapy, pharmacotherapy, or both ?

Many people benefit from a combined approach:

- **Psychotherapy first line** for depressive and anxiety symptoms related to chronic illness, body image disturbance, or poor coping (CBT, ACT, and specialized body-image work).
- **Medications** (antidepressants, anxiolytics) are appropriate when symptoms are moderate-to-severe, when rapid symptom control is necessary (e.g., severe insomnia or suicidal ideation), or when therapy alone is not sufficient. Antidepressants can also improve sleep and pain in some cases. Medication decisions are best made in collaboration with a psychiatrist or a primary-care clinician with psychopharmacology experience.
- **Integrated care** (therapist + prescriber + specialist team) often yields the best results for people facing complex medical and psychological needs.

If you're unsure, a good first step is a mental-health screening (PHQ-9 for depression, GAD-7 for anxiety) with your primary care or specialist; scores can guide the urgency of referral.

Supporting a loved one with lipedema — practical tips for families and partners

Caregivers and partners want to help but often worry about saying the wrong thing. Here's a short guide:

1. **Listen and validate.** "That sounds really hard." Validation reduces shame and opens doors.
2. **Avoid solution-only talk.** Saying "just diet and exercise" minimizes the lived experience. If you have ideas, ask permission: "Would you like help brainstorming?"
3. **Offer practical help.** Assist with logistics after surgery, go with them to a compression fitting, or help research reputable clinicians.
4. **Encourage professional help when needed.** Gently suggest therapy if you notice withdrawal, self-harm signals, or persistent despair. Offer to help find a therapist or join a first appointment for support.
5. **Set boundaries and practice self-care.** Caring for someone with a chronic condition is emotionally demanding; family members also benefit from support and, when needed, their own therapy.

Navigating the healthcare system — advocacy and communication tips

Poor clinician communication and dismissal are common sources of trauma in lipedema care. Here are practical ways to improve appointments:

- **Bring a one-page symptom timeline** (on paper or phone) that lists onset, treatments tried, and the biggest current problems.
- **Bring a family member or friend** for support and to help remember details.
- **Ask targeted questions**: "What do you think is driving my pain?" "What conservative therapies should I try for three months before reconsidering surgery?" "Can you screen me for anxiety/depression or refer me to a mental-health clinician experienced in chronic disease?"
- **If dismissed, seek a second opinion.** Many experienced lipedema clinics exist, and a second opinion often changes the course of care.

Good clinicians listen; poor experiences are not your fault.

Special topics

Eating disorders and "anorexic lipedema"

Some people with lipedema develop disordered eating from prolonged shame and the desperate belief that extreme weight loss will remove limb fat. If you struggle with restrictive eating, bingeing, or purging, you need specialized care: an eating-disorder therapist, medical monitoring, and a coordinated plan that addresses both lipedema and disordered eating simultaneously. This is a high-priority red flag and should prompt urgent referral. (Prevalence estimates vary; clinicians report higher than general population rates.)

Post-surgical psychological adjustment

Surgery can bring euphoria and relief, but patients sometimes experience unexpected emotional ups and downs during recovery (body image shifts, dependency stress). Preoperative counseling — even a single session — that outlines likely emotional reactions improves outcomes. Peer groups with postsurgical members also help normalize the roller coaster.

Building a personalized psychological care plan — a template

1. **Screening (baseline):** PHQ-9, GAD-7, sleep inventory, brief body-image questionnaire.
2. **Short-term goals (0–3 months):** Treat acute distress (sleep, pain coping), begin CBT or ACT, connect to a peer group, start a pacing plan.
3. **Medium goals (3–9 months):** Strengthen coping skills, address body image and relationship concerns, increase activity tolerance, review need for medication.
4. **Long term (9+ months):** Maintain skills, plan for periodic "booster" therapy sessions around major life events or surgical stages, continue peer-support engagement.

This flexible plan puts mental-health care on the same timetable as medical care.

Practical resources — where to begin

(Choose the one that fits you: clinician referral, a reliable organization, or a moderated peer group. Below are starting points clinicians and patients commonly use.)

- Cleveland Clinic — patient resources on lipedema and referral options.
- American Psychological Association — finder for licensed psychologists and resources on evidence-based therapies like CBT.
- National Institute of Mental Health — authoritative guides on depression, anxiety, and finding treatment.
- Local and national lipedema organizations and moderated support groups (search regional advocacy groups for vetted, evidence-minded communities). Peer communities can be found through specialty clinics and national organizations.

Final thoughts — compassion, courage, and a plan.

Living well with lipedema means caring for the whole person. The physical interventions — compression, physiotherapy, liposuction — often help in dramatic ways. But mental-health care is the engine that converts those physical gains into sustainable life change. It's not a moral failure to need psychological support; it's an intelligent, evidence-based step that most people with chronic conditions take.

Start small: one trusted clinician, one short therapy trial, one peer meeting. Build a support network that includes medical, physical, and psychological experts. Treat yourself with the same respect you'd offer a close friend in pain: listen, validate, and then plan the next step together.

Chapter 11 — Lifestyle Modifications

Living with lipedema is a long game — not a single treatment or quick fix. The everyday choices you make about food, movement, sleep, stress, social connection, and how you organize your life matter a great deal. This chapter gathers the evidence and the practical wisdom into a compassionate, doable playbook: why lifestyle changes help, which ones are high-yield, how to make them stick, and how to protect your mental health while doing the work. Where clinical evidence exists, I'll cite it; where it doesn't, I'll give sensible, harm-minimizing guidance informed by best practice.

Why lifestyle modifications matter (and what they can — and cannot — do)

First, an honest framing: lifestyle changes are **not** a cure for the abnormal fat of lipedema. Lipedema fat is biologically different and often resistant to diet-only approaches. However, lifestyle changes are powerful allies: they reduce inflammation and pain, protect lymphatic and venous function, improve sleep and mood, lower the risk of metabolic and cardiovascular disease, and make conservative and surgical treatments work better. In short — they don't erase lipedema, but they change the lived experience in meaningful ways. This approach is supported by multidisciplinary clinical guidance recommending compression, exercise, nutrition, and psychological care as core parts of ongoing management.

The five pillars of a lipedema-friendly lifestyle

Think of your life like a house: when the foundation is solid, individual renovations (surgery, new compression, a physiotherapy program) hold better. The five pillars below are the foundation.

1. Nutrition that reduces inflammation and supports metabolic health.
2. Movement that activates the muscle pump, preserves joints, and increases function.
3. Compression and lymph-supportive habits to contain swelling and protect tissues.
4. Sleep, stress management, and recovery — the often-overlooked restorers.
5. Psychological and social care — peer support, therapy, and practical advocacy.

Each pillar interacts with the others: good sleep helps exercise recovery; reduced inflammation from diet lowers pain and makes movement easier; strong social support reduces shame and increases adherence.

Pillar 1 — Nutrition: practical, evidence-informed strategies

What we eat affects inflammation, circulation, and how our body feels. Research into lipedema nutrition is growing and points toward anti-inflammatory patterns (Mediterranean-style, whole-food, or individualized low-carb approaches) as useful frameworks rather than miracle diets. The goal is symptom reduction, better energy, and metabolic health — not an expectation that limb shape will fully normalize by dieting alone.

Actionable nutrition plan

- **Prioritize whole foods.** Vegetables (especially leafy greens), berries, nuts, seeds, legumes (if tolerated), and whole grains or lower-glycemic alternatives form the base.
- **Omega-3s as a regular habit.** Fatty fish (salmon, mackerel, sardines) twice weekly or a high-quality fish oil supplement can reduce inflammatory signals for many people.
- **Reduce ultra-processed foods and added sugars.** These foods increase systemic inflammation and fluid shifts for susceptible people.
- **Salt sensitivity:** for some people, lowering sodium reduces transient fluid retention. Monitor blood pressure and symptoms; don't over-restrict sodium without medical advice.
- **Personalize carbohydrate amounts.** Some people benefit from a moderate-carb Mediterranean approach; others find symptom improvements with structured lower-carb or ketogenic patterns for limited periods. Work with a clinician if you have diabetes, kidney disease, or plan a strict regimen.
- **Meals that stabilize energy:** include protein + healthy fat + fiber at each meal to avoid blood sugar spikes that can worsen fatigue and cravings.

Supplements — useful but not required

- **Omega-3 fatty acids** (EPA/DHA): evidence supports anti-inflammatory effects.
- **Vitamin D** if deficient — check levels and replace as needed.

- **Curcumin (bioavailable forms)** has plausible anti-inflammatory benefits for some people; discuss with your clinician about interactions (especially with blood thinners).

Practical habits to start today

- Replace a sugary drink with water or herbal tea.
- Add one more vegetable serving to two meals per day for a week.
- Try a fatty fish meal twice this week or a daily fish-oil capsule (after checking with your clinician).

Pillar 2 — Movement: the anti-pain, pro-function prescription

Movement is medicine — especially for lipedema. The point is not punishment or rapid weight loss; it's activating the muscle pump, improving circulation, and building strength so daily life gets easier. Evidence supports low-impact, regular activity (walking, aquatic exercise, cycling) combined with targeted strength and mobility training. When exercise is combined with compression and lymphatic care, outcomes are better.

Key principles

- **Start gentle, progress slowly.** Begin with frequent short sessions (10–15 minutes) and increase duration weekly.
- **Prioritize low-impact aerobic activity** — walking, water workouts, stationary cycling — to maximize muscle pump without stressing joints.

- **Add resistance training 2×/week** focusing on functional strength: sit-to-stand, hip bridges, rows, step-ups. Strength helps posture and reduces joint pain.
- **Include mobility, breathing, and core work** (Pilates, gentle yoga) to support posture and lymphatic flow.
- **Use compression during exercise** if it helps comfort and containment; get garments fitted by a specialist.

Sample weekly plan (flexible)

- 3–4 days of 30–45 minutes walking or water exercise (can be split).
- 2 days of 20–30 minutes functional strength work.
- Daily 5–10 minutes of diaphragmatic breathing and gentle self-MLD (if trained).

Progression rules

- Increase total activity time by no more than 10% per week.
- Use symptom tracking: if pain or swelling increases and does not settle in 48–72 hours, reduce load and consult your therapist.

Practical tips

- Choose activities you enjoy—social exercise beats solitary boredom.
- Use a step counter or simple calendar to reinforce consistency.
- Work with a physiotherapist familiar with lipedema when possible.

Pillar 3 — Compression & lymph-supportive daily habits

Compression is a cornerstone conservative therapy. When used consistently and correctly, garments reduce pain and improve function during the day; combined with exercise and lymphatic care they produce better outcomes. Evidence supports compression use tailored to stage and limb shape, and combined compression+exercise programs show better results than exercise alone.

Practical guidance

- **Get professionally fitted.** Off-the-shelf garments often fit poorly; a certified fitter can recommend round-knit vs flat-knit and the right compression class.
- **Wear during prolonged standing, exercise, and travel.** Many people use daytime garments and remove them for sleep unless advised otherwise.
- **Rotate garments and care for them properly.** Have at least two sets for daily wear; replace every 6–12 months as elasticity declines.
- **Combine compression with MLD or self-MLD.** Lymphatic drainage (manual or self-applied) plus compression accelerates fluid movement and reduces fibrosis risk.

Daily micro-habits

- Elevate legs for 10–20 minutes after long standing to reduce pooling.
- Move every 30–60 minutes during prolonged sitting (even a 2-minute walk).
- Maintain skin hygiene and quick treatment of any breaks to prevent cellulitis.

Pillar 4 — Sleep, stress reduction, and recovery

Sleep and stress aren't "nice extras" — they fundamentally change pain sensitivity, inflammation, and decision-making. Poor sleep increases pain and reduces ability to exercise and stick to nutrition plans. Chronic stress elevates inflammatory signaling. Prioritizing recovery is as medically useful as compression or exercise.

Sleep basics

- **Consistent sleep schedule:** same bedtime and wake time 7 days/week.
- **Bedroom hygiene:** dark, cool, quiet environment; limit screens 60 minutes before bed.
- **Address sleep disorders:** if you snore heavily or feel unrefreshed, get evaluated for sleep apnea or insomnia; CBT-I is the first-line treatment for chronic insomnia.

Stress management techniques

- **Brief daily practices:** 5–10 minutes of diaphragmatic breathing, mindfulness, or progressive muscle relaxation.
- **Movement as medicine:** a short walk or gentle yoga session can lower cortisol and improve mood.
- **Pacing:** plan activities around energy windows to avoid boom-and-bust cycles that worsen pain and fatigue.

Recovery scheduling

- Build weekly "green zones" with low-demand days for physical and cognitive rest.
- Use a simple journal to spot patterns: which activities consistently cause a delayed flare-up?

Pillar 5 — Psychological care, social connection, and advocacy

Lipedema carries a heavy emotional load: shame, misdiagnosis, isolation, and grief are common. Psychological care and peer support are treatments, not luxuries. Addressing mental health improves treatment adherence and quality of life.

Concrete steps

- **Screen for mood and anxiety.** Use simple tools (PHQ-9, GAD-7) with your primary care provider and ask for referrals if scores are elevated. Evidence shows higher rates of emotional disturbance in lipedema populations; integrating mental-health care into routine management is recommended.
- **Therapy options:** CBT for pain and mood, ACT for acceptance and values work, and body-image therapies as needed. Group therapy or psychoeducation groups are particularly helpful for stigma and social isolation.
- **Peer support:** join moderated lipedema or lymphedema groups run by reputable organizations—peer connection reduces isolation and supplies practical tips that save months of trial-and-error.
- **Advocacy and empowerment:** learning to speak to clinicians clearly (symptom timelines, specific questions) increases the chance of good care. Preparing a one-page history and goals for appointments is often transformative.

Red flags — when to get urgent help

- Persistent suicidal thoughts, severe functional decline, uncontrolled eating-disorder behaviors, or substance misuse require immediate professional attention.

Putting it together: creating a sustainable lifestyle plan

A sustainable plan doesn't demand perfection. It asks for consistency and kindness.

Step-by-step 12-week starter plan

1. **Weeks 0–2 — Foundations:** pick one nutrition swap (e.g., replace sugary drinks with water), start daily 10–15 minute walks, order compression garment fitting, begin diaphragmatic breathing each morning and evening.
2. **Weeks 3–6 — Build habit & structure:** increase walks to 20–30 minutes 3×/week or start water exercise; add two 20-minute strength sessions; schedule an initial session with a physiotherapist or lymph therapist; join a peer support group.
3. **Weeks 7–12 — Integrate & personalize:** refine nutrition (increase vegetables, add two omega-3 meals/week), tailor exercise based on symptom response, begin 10–15 minutes daily self-MLD if taught, and schedule a mental-health screening or first therapy visit if needed.

Use a simple tracking sheet: energy, pain (0–10), minutes of activity, compression worn (yes/no), and one mood rating. Small, consistent changes compound.

Practical barriers and solutions

Barrier: cost of compression, therapy, or PT.
Solution: ask about charity grants, insurer coverage (some recognize lipedema care), community low-cost clinics, or staged purchases (one garment, then a second).

Barrier: low motivation due to pain/depression.
Solution: start with 5 minutes of activity, buddy up with a friend, or do a single meaningful task each day to build success.

Barrier: conflicting or extreme advice online.
Solution: prefer sources tied to multidisciplinary clinics, peer organizations that cite the literature, or clinical guidelines. If unsure, ask your clinician to help appraise the source.

Lifestyle and surgical care — the best partnership

If you choose surgery for symptom reduction, lifestyle habits remain essential both before and after. Good nutrition and controlled weight reduce surgical risk; prehab (moderate exercise and breathing training) speeds recovery; post-op compression, MLD, and a graded exercise program protect outcomes. Centers that integrate lifestyle programs into surgical pathways report better patient satisfaction and fewer complications.

Quick reference — daily checklist (printable)

- Drink water (aim for your usual hydration target).
- Eat 3 balanced meals with vegetables + protein + healthy fat.
- Move 20–30 minutes (walking, water exercise, or cycling).
- Wear compression during activity or prolonged standing (if fitted).

- Do 5–10 minutes diaphragmatic breathing + brief self-MLD (if trained).
- Sleep routine: consistent bedtime/wake time.
- Reach out to a peer or support contact once this week.

Resources and where to learn more

Trusted clinical summaries and recent reviews are helpful starting points for patients and clinicians; examples include multidisciplinary guidance and patient resources that synthesize the best current evidence on compression, exercise, nutrition, and combined conservative care. For summaries and clinical reading, see major guidelines and review resources.

Final thoughts — compassion, persistence, and personalization

Lifestyle change for lipedema is a marathon of small, meaningful choices rather than a single dramatic change. The work can feel relentless, but it pays real dividends: less pain, more movement, better sleep, and higher quality of life. Start where you are, prioritize one change, measure how it affects your symptoms and energy, and build from there. Treat yourself like a collaborator in your care — curious, evidence-seeking, and clear about your goals. With realistic expectations and a support team, lifestyle adjustments become a source of empowerment rather than another punishment.

Chapter 12 — Patient Stories and Case Studies

Hearing other people's stories does more than inform — it humanizes medical facts and turns abstract diagnostics into living decisions. In this chapter I share two detailed patient journeys: one that shows how community and connection transform isolation into strength, and another that shows how individual advocacy can change public conversation and policy. After each story I unpack clinical lessons, psychosocial implications, and practical care plans clinicians and patients can use. Where helpful, I link to published evidence showing these experiences are common and not anecdotal.

Angelique — From isolation to community

The arc of her story (summary)

Angelique's journey began early: subtle disproportion of the lower body in childhood, years of being mislabelled "overweight" or told she was simply lazy, and a long wait for a clinician who would listen and give a name to her symptoms. That misdiagnosis produced shame, secrecy, and a cycle of trying extreme diets that never changed the disproportionate leg fat — while pain, bruising, and mobility problems quietly worsened. Eventually she found peer support online and at a specialist clinic; that combination of knowledge and belonging remade how she approached care.

Her life did not become perfect, but her sense of agency did: she learned to pair evidence-based conservative care with psychological support and to become a trusted voice in her regional peer network. Her experience mirrors many documented trajectories in the literature: delayed diagnosis, psychological burden, and dramatic gains from multidisciplinary care and social support.

What happened and why it mattered

- **A long diagnostic delay.** Like many patients, Angelique's early signs were minimized. Research shows that misdiagnosis and long diagnostic journeys are common in lipedema and are major drivers of psychological distress.
- **Self-directed trial treatments.** Repeated dieting and exercise plans focused on weight loss rather than symptom control increased shame and fatigue — a frequent pattern in qualitative studies of lived experience.

- **Community as treatment.** The social support she found — online forums, local meetups, and a patient-led education group — served three therapeutic functions: they reduced isolation, delivered practical tips (compression brands, trusted therapists), and modeled reasonable expectations for care and outcomes. Studies consistently find that social support improves coping and lowers perceived stigma in lipedema.

A reconstructed care plan (what clinicians did with Angelique)

Below is a practical, staged plan modeled on how many specialists treat similar patients. It's written so a clinician and patient can discuss and adapt it.

1. **Comprehensive reassessment (week 0):**
    - Full history emphasizing onset at life stages (puberty, pregnancy), bruising tendency, pain, and family history.
    - Focused physical exam documenting distribution, Stemmer sign, pitting, and tissue texture.
    - Baseline questionnaires: PHQ-9, GAD-7, and a validated quality-of-life measure (e.g., SF-36 or disease-specific scale). Evidence shows these tools capture the psychological burden commonly seen.
2. **Conservative therapy initiation (weeks 0–12):**
    - Compression garment fitting (flat-knit when limb shapes are irregular), instruction on wear time and care.
    - Begin supervised, low-impact exercise program (aquatic therapy + progressive walking) with PT trained in lymphatic awareness.

- Start manual lymphatic drainage (MLD) once wounds/infections are excluded; teach simple self-MLD for daily use.
- Diet referral for an anti-inflammatory plan focused on symptom control rather than extreme weight loss.

3. **Psychosocial supports (concurrent):**
   - Brief CBT focusing on pacing, shame-reframing, and behavioral activation. CBT is effective for chronic illness–related distress.
   - Peer group connection and referral to a trusted advocacy organization for practical resources (compression funding, surgical info). Peer connection is an evidence-backed buffer against isolation.

4. **Surgical evaluation (after 6–12 months if refractory):**
   - If pain and functional limits persist despite optimized conservative care, evaluate candidacy for lymph-sparing liposuction at an experienced center. Prehab (exercise and nutrition optimization) and clear shared expectations are critical.

5. **Measures and follow-up:**
   - Track symptom scores (pain scales, activity minutes), PHQ-9/GAD-7, garment adherence, and any infections (cellulitis). Reassess every 3 months. Research shows longitudinal monitoring captures improvements in QoL and mental health over time.

Clinical lessons from Angelique's case

- **Don't blame the patient.** Early dismissal is common and causes avoidable psychological harm — clinicians should assume best intent and test for lipedema when distribution, bruising, and tenderness are present.

- **Integrate mental health early.** Screening and early referral to CBT or supportive counseling improve adherence to conservative care plans.
- **Peer groups are clinical allies.** They reduce isolation and speed practical learning (where to get garments, how to find good therapists). Encourage vetted peer resources rather than discouraging all online support.

Kasi — Advocacy through personal health

The arc of her story (summary)

Kasi's journey shows how personal narrative can become public advocacy. After living with lipedema for years and experiencing the frustration of misdiagnosis, she went public with a heartfelt social-media post that resonated widely. That visibility turned into a mission: public talks, podcast appearances, and work with patient organizations to normalize conversations about chronic health and reduce stigma.

Her message emphasizes dignity, practical self-care, and social responsibility: health differences don't diminish worth or potential. Her path illustrates how individual advocacy helps expand public knowledge and can even influence clinical empathy. Her public presence reflects many documented examples where patient advocates accelerate awareness and improve help-seeking behavior among peers.

What happened and why it mattered

- **From private struggle to public voice.** Kasi's disclosure created community ripple effects: others reached out, clinicians learned from patient feedback, and advocacy groups amplified her message. Patient narratives are powerful drivers of awareness and can reduce time to diagnosis for others.
- **Stigma-reduction and education.** Her work targeted two audiences: the public (normalizing diverse bodies) and clinicians (encouraging listening and upstream referral). Studies show education and exposure to patient narratives reduce stigmatizing attitudes among clinicians.

A reconstructed advocacy + care pathway (what worked for Kasi and could help others)

Here's a reproducible framework that clinicians and patient advocates can use together.

1. **Personal stabilization (months 0–6):**
   - Clinical optimization: ensure compression, MLD access, and a basic exercise/nutrition plan. It's easier to advocate effectively when symptoms are controlled well enough to sustain public work.
   - Psychological support: peer and professional support to process public disclosure and manage boundary setting.
2. **Strategic storytelling (months 6–12):**
   - Develop clear, evidence-grounded personal narratives (what happened, what helped, what was harmful). Use patient-story templates that include medical facts and actionable resources. Research shows framing stories around care pathways helps clinicians see where systems fail.
3. **Partnership with organizations (ongoing):**

- Collaborate with reputable advocacy groups to amplify accurate information and avoid misinformation. This increases credibility and reach.
4. **Clinician education and system change:**
    - Use patient panels, short recorded testimonials for clinics, and joint patient-clinician workshops to reduce diagnostic delay and stigma. Evidence supports inter-professional education involving patients as a method to change behavior.
5. **Monitoring impact:**
    - Track metrics: increased referrals to lipedema clinics, reduced average diagnostic delay (if data available), social-media engagement metrics tied to resources (garment suppliers, PT referrals). Advocacy gains traction when linked to measurable system changes.

Clinical and public-health lessons from Kasi's case

- **Patient voices change systems.** Individual advocacy can accelerate awareness, reduce stigma, and improve patient pathways when coupled with evidence and organizational partnerships.
- **Support advocates clinically.** Clinicians and health systems should offer anticipatory guidance to patients who plan public disclosure: ensure their symptoms and mental health are addressed before advocacy escalates.
- **Measure advocacy outcomes.** Simple metrics (referral numbers, website resource hits) show whether messaging helps or creates confusion; this enables rapid correction and quality control.

Two short clinical case studies (condensed, evidence-based)

Case A — "Early stage, heavy emotions"

- **Profile:** 32-year-old female, gradual bilateral thigh enlargement since puberty, pain on palpation, easy bruising, BMI 26, negative Stemmer sign. Symptoms worsen with pregnancy. PHQ-9 = 10 (moderate).
- **Plan:** confirm diagnosis clinically + ultrasound to exclude venous disease; start compression (round-knit initially), refer to physiotherapy for aquatic exercise and self-MLD, dietitian consult for anti-inflammatory plan, 8 weekly CBT sessions targeting body image and pacing; reassess at 3 months.
- **Rationale:** Early conservative management reduces symptom burden and prevents secondary lymphatic overload; early CBT addresses depression that impairs adherence. Evidence shows early, multidisciplinary care improves QoL.

Case B — "Refractory pain, considering surgery"

- **Profile:** 48-year-old female, long history of lipedema with progressive lobular fat and frequent cellulitis, tried conservative care for 2 years with partial response. Persistent functional limitation. PHQ-9 = 6 (mild).

- **Plan:** multidisciplinary surgical evaluation for staged lymph-sparing liposuction at an experienced center; prehab (6–8 weeks) including optimized nutrition, compression education, and preoperative MLD; post-op plan includes continuous compression, MLD, VTE prophylaxis, and a 12-week graded rehab program. Long-term plan: continued compression and mental-health follow-up.

Common themes across stories and studies (what the literature confirms)

1. **The psychological burden is high.** Multiple reviews and primary studies show elevated rates of depression, anxiety, and decreased QoL in people with lipedema. Routine screening and integrated care are recommended.
2. **Diagnostic delay is tragic and fixable.** Misdiagnosis fuels shame and harms outcomes. Education for primary care clinicians shortens the pathway to correct diagnosis.
3. **Peer and advocacy work improves access and resilience.** Patient stories on platforms and organized advocacy increase awareness and reduce isolation; partnering with reputable organizations channels enthusiasm into safe, evidence-based resources.
4. **Multidisciplinary care is best practice.** Combining compression, physiotherapy, nutrition, mental-health supports, and surgical options when indicated produces the best functional and psychological outcomes.

Practical tools for clinicians and patients

- **One-page symptom timeline:** a simple sheet that lists onset, precipitating events, prior treatments and responses, and family history — invaluable for first specialty visits. (Use the sample in Chapter 9 as a template.)
- **Screening bundle:** PHQ-9, GAD-7, and a short QoL tool at baseline and every 3 months for at least the first year of care. Evidence supports this interval for tracking change.
- **Peer-group directory:** maintain a vetted list of patient organizations and moderated online groups to recommend; encourage patients to sample and report back which groups felt safe and practical.

Closing reflections — stories as clinical compass

Angelique and Kasi show two complementary truths: personal healing and public change are possible. Angelique's recovery arc highlights the clinical and psychosocial gains of integrated care and peer belonging; Kasi's advocacy shows how individual voices shift culture and practice. The research confirms both patterns: the psychological burden is substantial, but targeted, multidisciplinary care — augmented by community and advocacy — reduces suffering and shortens the path to effective treatment. For clinicians: listen first, screen routinely, offer multidisciplinary plans, and partner with reputable patient groups. For patients: your story matters — to your care team, to peers, and to the system. Sharing it, with safety and boundaries, helps others find the care you wished you'd had sooner.

CONCLUSION

Future Directions in Lipedema Treatment

The field of lipedema research is burgeoning, with significant strides made in recent years. More than half of all studies on lipedema have been published in the last few years, indicating a growing interest and understanding of the condition. Researchers are now focusing on improving the quality of life for those with lipedema, exploring the different types of pain associated with the condition, and investigating the role of the immune system in lipedema pain. These promising leads could pave the way for new treatments and a better understanding of lipedema.

Empowering Patients for Self-Management

Empowerment is key in managing a chronic condition like lipedema. Tailored compression garment regimens and patient education are crucial tools for self-management. By equipping patients with the necessary knowledge and practical support, healthcare professionals can help improve outcomes and enhance the quality of life for those living with lipedema. Additionally, embracing oneself and engaging in self-care activities such as yoga or meditation can build confidence and reduce the shame associated with physical symptoms. Empowerment comes from within, and with the right tools and support, patients can take control of their lipedema management.

In conclusion, Lipedema Solution serves as a comprehensive guide for those affected by lipedema. It provides practical advice on managing the condition through compression therapy, diet, and surgical options. The book also emphasizes the importance of psychological support, lifestyle modifications, and the power of patient stories. As we look to the future, we see a landscape where patients are empowered, treatments are evolving, and hope is on the horizon. Together, we can continue to improve the lives of those living with lipedema.

IF YOU VALUES FROM THIS BOOK DO WELL TO DROP A POSITIVE REVIEW FOR ME.

YOU CAN ALSO CHECK MY OTHER BOOKS HERE....
https://www.amazon.com/author/elvygraves